Contemporary News in Health and Community by Basic English

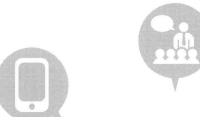

やさしい英語ニュースで学ぶ
現代社会と健康

Yoshifumi Tanaka
田中芳文
［編著］

講談社

執筆者一覧

飯島睦美
群馬大学大学教育・学生支援機構大学教育センター　教授　　　　　　　　　　　　　(13)

岩田　淳
島根大学医学部　教授　　　　　　　　　　　　　　　　　　　　　　　　　(2, 7)

片岡由美子
愛知県立大学看護学部　准教授　　　　　　　　　　　　　　　　　　　　　(3, 4)

ケン・スレイマン
天使大学看護栄養学部　准教授　　　　　　　　　　　　　　　　　　　（英文校正）

※田中芳文
島根県立大学人間文化学部　教授　　　　　　　　　　　　　　　(5, 6, 10, 15)

廣渡太郎
日本赤十字秋田看護大学看護学部　教授　　　　　　　　　　　　　　　　　　(9)

マユーあき
島根県立大学人間文化学部　教授　　　　　　　　　　　　　　　　　　　(8, 12)

山内　圭
新見公立大学健康科学部　教授　　　　　　　　　　　　　　　　　　　　　(14)

山﨑麻由美
神戸常盤大学保健科学部　教授　　　　　　　　　　　　　　　　　　　　(1, 11)

五十音順、※は編著者。（　）内の数字は担当Unit。

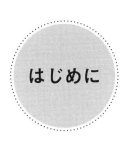

はじめに

　超高齢化社会を迎えた今，健康は私たち現代人の重要な関心事となっています。本書は，VOA（Voice of America）でとりあげられた現代社会と健康に関するニュースを読みながら英語を学習するためのテキストです。全部で15のUnitに出てくる主なキーワードは，子どもの発育，食生活，アルツハイマー病，睡眠，喫煙，子宮頸がん，脊髄損傷，有害化学物質，大気汚染，認知症，性犯罪，過労死，肥満，医療費，麻薬といったものです。

　なるべく辞書を引かなくても読み進めることができるように，英文にはできる限り多くの脚注が付けてあります。Unit 1～4, 6～9, 11～14の練習問題は，A（内容理解），B（書き取り），C（英文整序），D（語彙）から構成されています。また，Unit 5, 10, 15は，少し構成を変えて，適語補充，英文整序，英文和訳，語彙の練習問題に加えて，それ以前の4つのUnitに出てきた重要表現・構文・語彙の復習ができるように工夫しました。

　本書を利用することによって，「現代社会と健康」に関するみなさんの知識が深まると同時に，英語の学力が向上することを願っています。

　最後に，本書出版の意義にご理解をいただいた講談社サイエンティフィクに敬意を表しますとともに，前書『英文ニュースで学ぶ　健康とライフスタイル』に引き続き出版のためにご尽力くださった同社の小笠原弘高さんにこころより感謝申し上げます。

2017年初秋

編著者

Contents

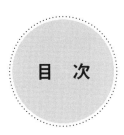
目 次

はじめに iii

Unit 1 子どもの発育発達に欠かせないもの

A Child's Growing Brain Needs Love as Much as Food track 01 1

Best Tool to Teach Baby Talk? Their Parents' Voice track 02 4

Unit 2 世界一健康な人たちが食べるもの

What the World's Healthiest People Eat track 04 8

Unit 3 運動はアルツハイマー病にも効果的

Exercise Good for Brain, Even for Those with Alzheimer's track 06 14

Unit 4 睡眠不足がもたらす健康被害

Are Sleep Problems a Growing Epidemic? track 08 21

Caffeine Found to Disrupt Internal Clock, Sleep Patterns track 09 24

Unit 5 +Review 喫煙に安全なレベルは存在するのか?

Study : There's No Safe Level of Smoking track 11 29

Review (Unit 1〜Unit 4) 32

Unit 6 アフリカの発展途上国における子宮頸がん対策

Cancer a Public Health Concern in Africa's Developing Countries track 12 34

WHO Stresses Value of Vaccine in Preventing Cervical Cancer track 13 37

Unit 7 脊髄損傷の痛みを和らげる新しい手術

New Surgical Techniques Help Relieve Pain from Spinal Injury track 15 41

Unit 8 有害化学物質の行き着く先

Climate Change Could Increase Oceanic Mercury track 17 47

Fast Food Packaging Could Be Dangerous track 18 51

Unit 9 アジアの大都市が窒息⁉ 深刻化する大気汚染

Asian Cities Choking on Worsening Air Pollution track 20 56

Unit 10 +Review 認知症のリスクを下げるのは？

Strong Heart, Better Education Shown to Lower Dementia Risk track 22 64

Review （Unit 6 〜 Unit 9） 68

Unit 11 性犯罪のない大学をめざせ！

US Universities Work to Prevent Sexual Abuse track 23 70

Unit 12 生かされない教訓 日本の過労死問題

Japan Overwork Deaths Among Young Show Lessons Unlearned track 25 77

Unit 13 インドの肥満対策　ファーストフードに"肥満税"

India's Southern Kerala State Imposes "Fat Tax" on Fast Food track 27 ... 84

Unit 14 高騰するアジアの医療費　その原因は？

WHO, Medical Experts, Warn of Rising Health Costs in Asia track 29 91

Unit 15 ◆Review 麻薬使用に対する世界各国の取り組み

UN Hears Major Differences on Global Approach to Drug Use track 31 ... 98

　　　Review（Unit 11～Unit 14）.. 102

あらかじめご了承ください

・本書は全国の大学・専門学校で教材として使用されているため，練習問題の解答や日本語訳は付属していません。

・本書の紹介ページに，音声データが用意されています（収録箇所：各Unitの🔊の部分）。

紹介ページのアドレス
http://www.kspub.co.jp/book/detail/1556331.html

Unit 1 子どもの発育発達に欠かせないもの

A Child's Growing Brain Needs Love as Much as Food

Voice of America, July 04, 2016

track 01

Fewer babies and very young children are dying today compared to 20 years ago.

Over that period, the number of infant deaths has dropped sharply—from about 12 million to six million worldwide. Infant child mortality has been cut thanks to billions of dollars in aid and the work of many countries.

However, a group of experts say that is not enough. For children to grow and develop fully, they need more than a nutritious diet and access to medicine.

That is the opinion of a team of social scientists and public health experts. They found that about 200 million children are failing to meet their developmental potential each year. What is lacking, say the experts, is social interaction with the children and involvement by their caretakers.

The U.S. National Academy of Medicine set up the group of 32 academic experts. They provide strong evidence that just as a poor diet can harm children, violence and lack of care can damage a child's brain.

Notes:

compared to ～／～と比較すると　the number of ～／～の数　infant／幼児　mortality／死亡数, 死亡率　cut／減らす, 下げる　thanks to ～／～のおかげで　billions of ～／何十億もの～　aid／援助, 助成　expert／専門家　more than ～／～以上のもの　nutritious／栄養価の高い　diet／食事　access to ～／～を利用できること　medicine／医療　social scientist／社会科学者　public health／公衆衛生　fail to ～／～ができない　meet／到達する　developmental／発達の　potential／可能性, 見込み　what is lacking／不足しているもの　interaction／交流, ふれあい　involvement／関わり　caretaker／世話をする人　National Academy of Medicine／米国医学アカデミー（1970年設立の独立非営利団体）　set up ～／～を結成する　academic／学識ある　provide／提供する　evidence／証拠　just as ～／～と全く同じように　harm／害する　lack／不足

And that, they say, leads to physical and social stunting, even when aid programs are available. Stunting is when a person fails to grow and develop normally.

20　Neil Boothby is with the Mailman School of Public Health at Columbia University in New York. He likens social interaction to "investing in young children." He adds that "it's vital to ensuring international peace and security."

Boothby says that providing good, positive social interactions is as big a
25　part of development as providing food and water. And these positive social interactions must be consistent and not, what he calls, episodic.

He calls the wiring in the brain, circuitry. And he calls the structure of the brain, 'brain architecture.'

Here is Boothby.

30　"This becomes part of actually strengthening the circuitry in the brain. When the response isn't there, or it's episodically there, then that same circuitry, that same brain architecture is weakened. So it is not just micronutrient, it is also social care."

Boothby says studies have shown that international aid programs alone are not enough to help children reach their full ability.
35

Notes:

lead to ～／～をもたらす，～につながる　physical／身体的な　stunting／発達阻害　aid program／援助プログラム　available／利用できる　Mailman School of Public Health／メイルマン公衆衛生学部　Columbia University／コロンビア大学（米国ニューヨーク市にある私立大学）　liken A to B／AをBにたとえる　invest／投資する　add／付け加える　be vital to ～／～にとって必要不可欠な　ensure／確保する　security／安全　positive／前向きな　as ～ as .....／..... と同じくらい～である　consistent／首尾一貫した　what he calls／彼が言うところの　episodic／一時的な，気まぐれな　wiring／つながり　circuitry／回路　structure／構造　architecture／建築　strengthen／強化する　response／反応　episodically／偶発的に　weaken／弱める　not just A, also B／AだけでなくBも　micronutrient／（健全な成長に必要な)微量栄養素　～ alone／～だけで　enough to ～／～するのに十分である　reach／達する　ability／能力

The Columbia University researcher just returned from Uganda. In that country, he says, more than a third of the population suffers from stunting. Signs of stunting include smaller physical growth and lower than average scores on intelligence tests.

"For example, I met with some parents on this last trip. Fathers were saying, 'Ah, you know I don't really engage with the child until she or he is three months old because they're too little.' I mean that's counter to what they should be doing because holding, talking, caressing, etc., is all part of brain health."

The paper, says Boothby, is a call for social interaction to be added to the list of health and nutrition assistance programs and concerns.

"You know, we teach parents when they go to clinics about water and sanitation. We teach them about the kinds of foods children should eat. Why aren't we teaching them the things that make brains grow?"

Boothby adds it is time for international aid policies to catch up with scientific research. Aid policies, he says, must combine the neurobiology of caring with other forms of assistance.

Notes:

researcher／研究者 Uganda／ウガンダ（アフリカ東部の共和国） a third／三分の一 population／人口 suffer from〜／〜に苦しむ、〜を患う sign／徴候 include／含む physical growth／身体発育 average／平均の score／得点 intelligence test／知能検査 for example／例えば engage with〜／〜と関わる counter／逆の、反対の caress／愛撫する、なでる paper／研究論文 call／要請、要求 assistance program／援助プログラム concern／重要事項 clinic／外来診療所、クリニック sanitation／衛生設備 international aid policy／国際的援助政策 catch up with 〜／〜に追いつく combine A with B／AをBと結びつける neurobiology／神経生物学

Best Tool to Teach Baby Talk?   Their Parents' Voice

Voice of America, January 20, 2016

🔊 track 02

A new study says electronic toys are not helping babies learn.

"Even if companies are marketing them as educational, they're not teaching the babies anything at this time," said the study's author, Anna Sosa. She is a Northern Arizona University professor who heads the school's Child Speech and Language Lab.

Sosa and her fellow researchers listened to audio recordings of parents playing with their babies—aged 10 months to 16 months. The researchers compared the experiences when the children played with electronic toys, traditional toys such as blocks, or when the children looked at books.

What they found is that parents talked less with their babies when the babies played with electronic toys.

"The parents talked less, responded less and used fewer content specific words," Sosa said.

Why is this important?

Sosa said the research shows that how quickly children develop language is often based on what they hear from parents.

When the infants played with electronic toys, parents said little to their

Notes:
tool／道具　electronic／電子の　toy／おもちゃ, 玩具　even if ～／たとえ～だとしても　market A as B／AをBとして売り込む　educational／教育的な・ためになる　at this time／この時期には　author／執筆者　Northern Arizona University／北アリゾナ大学（米国アリゾナ州にある州立大学）　head／率いる　Child Speech and Language Lab／チャイルド・スピーチ・アンド・ランゲージ・ラボ（北アリゾナ大学のCommunication Sciences and Disorders学部内の研究所）　fellow researcher／仲間の研究者　audio recording／録音　aged ～／～の年齢の　compare／比較する　experiences／経験したこと　traditional／伝統的な, 昔ながらの　A such as B／Bのような A　less／より少なく　respond／答える　content word／内容語（名詞・形容詞・動詞・副詞のように内容を表す語）　specific／具体的な, 明確な　be based on ～／～に基づいている

children, Sosa said.

But with traditional toys, such as blocks, parents shared the names and descriptions of the animals, colors and shapes as their children played, Sosa said.

There was even more information given by parents as their babies looked at the pictures in books, Sosa said.

Sosa is not telling parents to throw out electronic toys. But she said parents should look at their infants' play with such toys as entertainment, not a learning experience.

Toy Industry Association spokeswoman Adrienne Appell responded to the study. She said it is important that parents make time to play with their children.

"Playing is a way that kids can learn so much, not only cognitive skills, but social and developmental skills," she said.

She added that play should be balanced, including time for just "make believe" activities, as well as traditional and electronic toys.

Notes:
share／共有する　description／描写　throw out 〜／〜を処分する　but 〜／（前の文のnotと呼応して）むしろ〜　look at A as B／AをBとみなす　entertainment／娯楽　learning experience／学習体験　Toy Industry Association／玩具産業協会（米国の非営利団体）　spokeswoman／広報担当者　make time to 〜／〜する時間を作る　way／方法　not only A but (also) B／Aだけでなく B も　cognitive／認知の　social／社会的な　"make believe" activity／「ごっこ」遊び／　A as well as B／BだけでなくAも

練習問題

A 本文の内容に合うように，各英文の（　）内に入るもっとも適切な語句をそれぞれ1つずつ選びなさい。

1. As well as a nutritious diet and access to medicine, children need (positive, complex, episodic) social interaction to fully grow and develop.
2. Neil Boothby says that international aid programs for children should include what helps their (skills, brains, relationships) develop.
3. According to Anna Sosa, children develop language from what they (study with, hear from, talk with) their parents.
4. Parents should look at electronic toys as (educational, traditional, entertaining) toys.

B 音声を聴いて，次の英文の（　）内に適語を記入しなさい。　　track 03

1. (　　) (　　) her tender care, the child soon got better.
2. The study (　　) (　　) (　　) careful experiments.
3. I'll (　　) (　　) (　　) you.
4. (　　) (　　) (　　) births is decreasing each year in Japan.

C 和文に合うように，（　）内の語句を並べかえて英文をつくりなさい。

1. 睡眠不足は万病の元になるかもしれない。
   (to, all, diseases, of, lead, lack, kinds of, may, sleep).

2. 何を食べるかだけでなく，どのようにして食べるかが大切だ。
   (important, only, is, how you eat, but also, not, what you eat).

3. 他者との社会的なふれあいは子どもの発達に不可欠である。
   (other people, to, interaction, is, a child's development, vital, with, social).

4. 誰もが良質な公共医療サービスを利用できるべきだ。
   (people, to, health services, should, good quality, access, all, have).

D 次の英語に相当する日本語を下から選び，記号で答えなさい。

1. play make-believe ( )　　2. fly a kite ( )
3. blow soap bubbles ( )　　4. play house ( )
5. do riddles ( )　　6. play hide-and-seek ( )
7. jump rope ( )　　8. play tag ( )
9. play with blocks ( )　　10. play musical chairs ( )

> a. かくれんぼをする　　b. なぞなぞ遊びをする　　c. 積み木遊びをする
> d. なわとびをする　　e. いすとり遊びをする　　f. しゃぼん玉を飛ばす
> g. ごっこ遊びをする　　h. ままごと遊びをする　　i. たこあげをする
> j. おにごっこをする

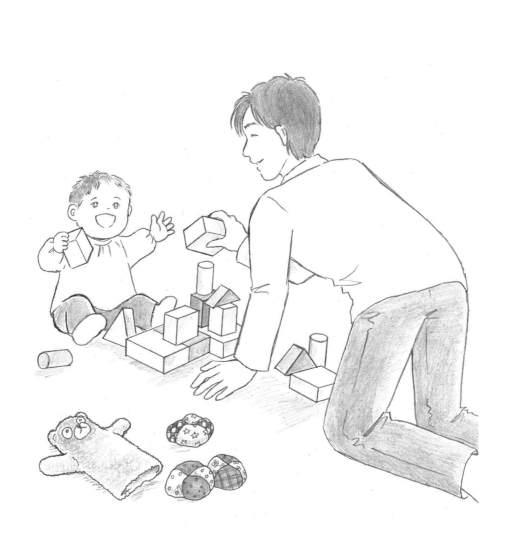

Unit 2 世界一健康な人たちが食べるもの

What the World's Healthiest People Eat

Voice of America, February 22, 2010

🔊 track 04

Everyday choices help prevent disease

Different foods, cooking techniques and lifestyles can explain why some people of some cultures are leaner, healthier and living longer than others. Dietitians and health experts say it's important to learn from the world's healthiest countries, if we want to lose weight, fight disease and enjoy a healthier life.

Healthiest Top 10

After years of traveling the globe, fitness expert Harley Pasternak has learned a lot about the diets and lifestyles of the world's healthiest countries. In his new book, *The 5-Factor World Diet*, he ranks the world's top 10 healthiest nations.

"The Japanese, in my opinion, are the healthiest population in the world," says Pasternak. "They have the longest lifespan in the world, the lowest incidence of obesity, heart disease and diabetes."

What and how the Japanese eat, he says, explains why they are the healthiest people on earth.

Notes:

prevent／予防する，防ぐ some people of some cultures 〜 than others／文化の異なる人たちと比べてより〜な人たちもいる（someに呼応するothersに注意） lean／痩せた dietitian／栄養士 expert／専門家 lose weight／体重を減らす（↔ gain weight） globe／世界 fitness／フィットネス（良好な健康状態） diet／食事 rank／ランク付けする in one's opinion／〜の意見では lifespan／寿命 incidence／発症率 obesity／（病的）肥満 diabetes／糖尿病 on earth／この世で，世界中で（最上級を強調）

"Every meal in Japan looks like a piece of art. Food is so beautiful and so delicious and so simple," says Pasternak. "They are the largest consumer of fish in the world and of whole soy and of seaweed and green tea. When they are about 80 percent full, they stop and wait for about 10 minutes, then decide whether to keep going. And most times, they are full so they don't need to keep eating more."

Three other Asian countries make Pasternak's top ten: Singapore, Korea and China. The list is rounded out by Israel, Sweden, France and two countries on the Mediterranean; Greece and Italy.

Mediterranean diet

"Italian food is extremely healthy from lentils and garbanzo beans to balsamic vinegars, small portions of homemade pastas," he explains. "They eat their largest meal of the day as lunch, not dinner. They have a big feast on Sundays. It's not a daily thing. They have something called *passeggiata*, so after every dinner they get up as a family and they go for a walk."

That Mediterranean diet is what cardiologist Richard Collins says he always recommends to his clients.

"The Mediterranean diet is very rich in vegetables and fruits and whole grains, lean meats and poultry, a lot of Omega 3 rich fish," says Collins. "And if you look at the lifestyle and eating style, they balance their physical activity with their calorie intake."

Collins is known as the Cooking Cardiologist. He says combining medical

---

Notes:

look like ～／～のように見える　a piece of art／芸術作品　consumer／消費者　whole soy／全粒大豆　seaweed／海藻　keep ～ing／～し続ける　round out ～／～を締めくくる　the Mediterranean／地中海　extremely／きわめて　lentil／レンズ豆　garbanzo bean／ひよこ豆　balsamic vinegar／バルサミコ酢　portion／(食事の)分量　feast／ごちそう　*passeggiata*／夕方の散歩　go for a walk／散歩に出かける　cardiologist／心臓病専門医, 循環器専門医　recommend／推奨する　be rich in ～／～が豊富な　whole grain／全粒穀物　lean meat／脂肪の(ほとんど)ない肉, 赤身の肉　poultry／鳥肉　Omega 3／オメガ3脂肪酸（体内のさまざまな機能にとって重要な不飽和脂肪酸）　balance A with B／AとBのバランスをとる　intake／摂取　be known as ～／～として知られている

and culinary expertise allows him to help people recognize the cooking mistakes that make their diet unhealthy.

"I think the first mistake is they start with unhealthy ingredients," he says. "They are not looking at the natural aspect of food. Number two, in looking at the cooking techniques, I've noticed we're tough on our food. We beat it up. We want it hot, we want it now, we want it deep fried, we want it blackened, we want it burnt. If you look at the European style of cooking, it's much more genteel: poaching, steaming, taking your time. We've got to realize that, because what happens when we're doing this to our food, we destroy essential vitamins."

Even small changes in what we eat and how we prepare our food can be very useful, says physician David Servan-Schreiber, author of *Anti-Cancer, A New Way of Life*.

"A recent study in China found that women who eat mushrooms three times a week have a 50 percent reduction in the risk of developing breast cancer. If they drink three cups of green tea, three times a week, they also have a 50 percent reduction in the risk of developing breast cancer," says Servan-Schreiber. "If they do both, they have an 89 percent reduction in the risk of developing breast cancer. So these are stunning numbers for something as simple as eating mushrooms and drinking green tea."

Spice of Life

Servan-Schreiber says people in countries that use lots of spices also experience better health. "Like turmeric, which is used in India very much, but also along with North African countries. And everywhere where people

Notes:

culinary／料理の　expertise／専門知識　allow A to ～／Aが～することを許す　start with ～／～で始める　ingredient／（料理の）材料　be tough on ～／～に厳しい態度で臨む　beat up ～／～を打ちのめす　deep fried／油で揚げた　blackened／黒い焦げ目がついた　burnt／真っ黒焦げになった　genteel／上品な　poach／ゆでる　steam／蒸す　take one's time／じっくり時間をかける　have got to ～／～しなければならない（= have to）　physician／医師　anti-cancer／抗がん　way of life／生き方　three times a week／週に3回　reduction／減少　breast cancer／乳がん　stunning／驚くほどの　as ～ as .....／.....と同じくらい～の　turmeric／ウコン　along with ～／～に加えて

use these spices and herbs—like thyme, rosemary, oregano, basil, mint and so on — the cancer rates are much lower, and when they have cancer, it's not as aggressive."

Physician Kelly Traver, author of *The Program: The Brain-Smart Approach to the Healthiest You*, agrees. She says knowledge about the world's healthiest diets has become more available than ever and can help us fight our worst enemy: obesity.

"What we've now learned is that fat is not just a deposit for energy in our bodies," says Traver. "Actually, each fat cell secretes at least 100 chemicals out of the cell into our bodies, which promote cancer, which promote aging, which promote inflammatory chemicals that can influence dementia, arthritis and heart disease. So, actually fat holds a bigger key in health, clearly, than just being a cosmetic issue."

Dietitians and health experts say understanding how important our food choices are, and learning a lesson or two from the world's healthiest nations, can help us live healthier, too.

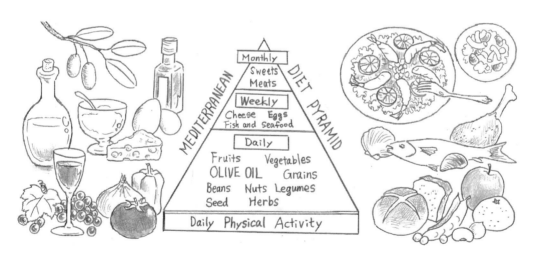

練習問題

A 本文の内容に合うように，各英文の（　）内に入るもっとも適当な語句をそれぞれ1つずつ選びなさい。

1. In his new book, fitness expert Harley Pasternak says the (Koreans, Chinese, Japanese) are the healthiest population in the world.
2. According to Richard Collins, known as the Cooking Cardiologist, we are not looking at the (poor, natural, unhealthy) aspect of food when cooking.
3. A study in China shows that eating mushrooms three times a week helps prevent women from developing (ovarian, breast, colon) cancer.
4. According to Kelly Traver, author of *The Program: The Brain-Smart Approach to the Healthiest You*, knowing more about the world's healthiest diets can help prevent (obesity, diabetes, stroke).

B 音声を聴いて，次の英文の（　）内に適語を記入しなさい。　　track 05

1. All patients (　　) (　　) and showed improvement in their metabolic syndrome.
2. The sky today (　　) (　　) a beautiful painting.
3. Pineapple juice (　　) (　　) (　　) vitamins A and B.
4. The doctor told me to take the medicine (　　) (　　) (　　) (　　) after every meal.

C 和文に合うように，（　）内の語句を並べかえて英文をつくりなさい。

1. ファイザー社（Pfizer）は世界で最も大きい製薬会社の1つです。
   (one, pharmaceutical, is, of, world's, companies, largest, the, Pfizer).

2. その奨学金のおかげで私は大学に行くことができた。
   (college, to, allowed, to, me, go, has, the scholarship).

3. 私たちが滞在したホテルは非常に便利で快適だった。
   (very, we, was, comfortable, the hotel, convenient, stayed, and, where).

4. 私たちが学校で学んだことは仕事を見つけるのに役立つでしょう。
   (what, us, help, we, find, at, learned, will, a job, to, school).

D 次の英語に相当する日本語を下から選び，記号で答えなさい。

1. calorie   ( )   2. dietician   ( )
3. intake   ( )   4. ingredient   ( )
5. portion   ( )   6. antioxidant   ( )
7. fiber   ( )   8. protein   ( )
9. carbohydrate   ( ) 10. lean   ( )

a. 繊維質   b. (肉が)脂肪分が少ない   c. (食事の)分量
d. タンパク質   e. カロリー   f. 栄養士
g. 炭水化物   h. (料理の)材料   i. 抗酸化物質
j. 摂取

Unit 3 運動はアルツハイマー病にも効果的

Exercise Good for Brain, Even for Those with Alzheimer's

Voice of America, July 27, 2015
Associated Press

🔊 track 06

WASHINGTON — Exercise may do more than keep a healthy brain fit: New research suggests working up a good sweat may also offer some help once memory starts to slide—and even improve life for people with Alzheimer's.

The effects were modest, but a series of studies reported last week found vigorous workouts by people with mild memory impairment decreased levels of a warped protein linked to risk of later Alzheimer's—and improved quality of life for people who already were in early stages of the disease.

"Regular aerobic exercise could be a fountain of youth for the brain," said cognitive neuroscientist Laura Baker of Wake Forest School of Medicine in North Carolina, who reported some of the research at the Alzheimer's Association International Conference.

Doctors have long advised that people keep active as they get older. Exercise is good for the heart, which in turn is good for the brain. Lots of research shows physical activity can improve cognition in healthy older

Notes:

Alzheimer's／アルツハイマー病（Alzheimer's disease）　Associated Press／AP通信社（世界的な通信網を持つ米国の大手通信社）　more than ～／～以上に　keep A fit／Aの健康を保つ　work up a good sweat／十分に汗をかく　once ～／いったん～すると　slide／徐々に悪化する　improve／改善する, 向上させる　effect／効果　modest／大きくない, そこそこの　a series of ～／一連の～　vigorous／精力的な　workout／トレーニング　impairment／障害　warped／ゆがんだ　protein／タンパク質　quality of life／生活の質（略語はQOL）　fountain of youth／若さの源泉　cognitive neuroscientist／認知神経科学者　Wake Forest School of Medicine／ウェイクフォレスト大学医学部（米国ノースカロライナ州にある私立大学）　the Alzheimer's Association International Conference／アルツハイマー病協会国際会議　in turn／次に, 同様にして　lots of ～／たくさんの～　cognition／認知力

people, potentially lowering their risk of developing dementia.

With no medications yet available that can slow Alzheimer's creeping brain destruction, the new findings point to lifestyle changes that might make a difference after memory impairment begins as well. The caveat: Check with a doctor to determine what's safe for a person's overall medical condition, especially if they already have Alzheimer's.

"It's important for caregivers especially to think how to keep loved ones as engaged as possible. The last thing they should do is keep their loved one at home watching TV," said Alzheimer's Association chief science officer Maria Carrillo.

How much exercise? In studies from North Carolina, Denmark and Canada, people got 45 minutes to an hour of aerobic exercise three or four times a week, compared to seniors who stuck with their usual schedule.

"You're panting and sweating," said Baker, whose research is getting particular attention because it's one of the first to find exercise can affect tau, an Alzheimer's hallmark that causes tangles in brain cells.

Baker studied 71 previously sedentary older adults who have hard-to-spot memory changes called mild cognitive impairment that can increase risk of developing Alzheimer's. They wore monitors to be sure the exercisers raised their heart rate enough and that the control group kept their heart rate deliberately low while doing simple stretch classes that allowed them to socialize.

Notes:

dementia／認知症　medication／薬物治療　available／利用できる　creeping／徐々に進行する　destruction／破壊　findings／（複数形で）研究結果　point to ～／～を指摘する　make a difference／重要である　～ as well／～もまた，そのうえ～も　caveat／警告　check with ～／～と相談する　overall／全体的な　loved one／最愛の人　as ～ as possible／できるだけ～　engaged／忙しい　the last thing ～／最も～でないこと　chief science officer／最高科学責任者　compared to ～／～と比べて　stick with ～／～に固執する，～をやり通す　pant／息切れする　sweat／汗をかく　affect／影響を及ぼす　tau (protein) ／タウ・タンパク質（中枢神経系および末梢神経系の神経細胞等に発現しているタンパク質）　hallmark／特徴　tangle／もつれ　previously／以前は　sedentary／座ってばかりいる　hard-to-spot／目立たない　heart rate／心拍数　control group／（実験の）対照群　deliberately ／故意に　allow A to ～／Aに～をさせる　socialize／社交活動をする

MRI scans showed the exercisers experienced increased blood flow in brain regions important for memory and thought processing—while cognitive tests showed a corresponding improvement in their attention, planning and organizing abilities, what scientists call the brain's "executive function," Baker reported.

Most intriguing, tests of spinal fluid also showed a reduction in levels of that worrisome tau protein in exercisers over age 70.

"This is really exciting," said Dr. Laurie Ryan of the National Institute on Aging. "It's too soon to say that lowers risk" of worsening memory, she cautioned, saying longer studies must test if sticking with exercise makes a lasting difference.

Later this year, Baker will begin a national study that will test 18 months of exercise in people with mild cognitive impairment.

Danish researchers reported last week that vigorous exercise prevented neuropsychiatric symptoms—aggression, irritability, delusions—in older adults with mild Alzheimer's.

Scientists at the University of Copenhagen studied 200 older adults for four months, and didn't find overall memory improvements, although the fraction that exercised the most intensely did see some improvement in their mental speed and attention.

But improving quality of life is important because those neuropsychiatric symptoms can complicate care dramatically and are one reason that

---

Notes:
MRI scan／MRI検査（磁気共鳴画像法による検査） blood flow／血流 region／領域 thought processing／思考処理 corresponding／それ相応の improvement／改善 organize／体系づける "executive function"／「実行機能」 intriguing／興味深い spinal fluid／(脳脊)髄液, 脊髄液 reduction／減少 worrisome／気にかかる, やっかいな the National Institute on Aging／米国国立老化研究所（略称はNIA） too ~ to .....／~すぎて.....できない lasting／永続的な prevent／防ぐ neuropsychiatric／精神神経系の symptom／症状 aggression／攻撃性 irritability／興奮性, 過敏性 delusion／妄想 the University of Copenhagen／コペンハーゲン大学（デンマーク最古の歴史を持つ大学） fraction／(全体からすると)ごく一部 complicate／複雑にする

dementia patients end up in nursing homes, said NIA's Ryan.

At the University of British Columbia, researchers studied 60 seniors with a different kind of mild memory impairment—caused by clogged arteries—and found six months of mostly treadmill exercise triggered improvements on cognitive tests.

Back in North Carolina, a participant in Baker's study said that learning to regularly exercise was challenging but he's glad he did. Michael Gendy, 62, said he'd never noticed memory problems before but now says he doesn't get tired as easily while climbing stairs, sleeps better and occasionally notices a little speedier memory.

"They helped me gear my mind toward how important it is," he said of continuing to keep active.

Baker said sedentary seniors can learn to exercise safely but they have to work up to it gradually, starting 10 minutes at a time.

"We baby these people," she said. "They're afraid of gyms. They don't have confidence in their own ability. We give them intensive one-on-one attention."

Gendy is trying to stick with his newfound exercise habits, taking a brisk evening walk or a bike ride despite the summer heat and signing up for occasional classes at the local YMCA.

"I'm going to keep on as long as I can, as long as my bones and my muscles and my brain can withstand all this," he said.

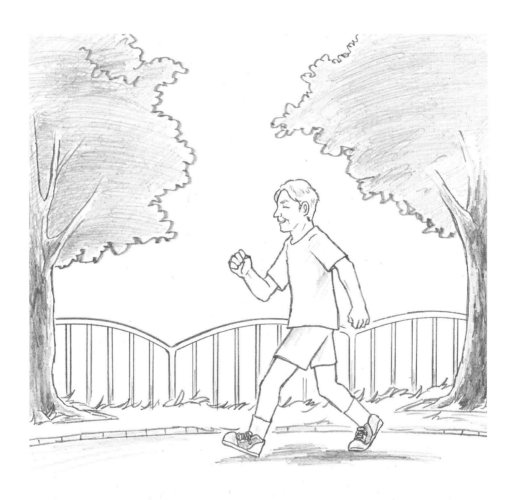

Notes:
withstand／耐える

練習問題

A 次の英文が本文の内容に一致する場合にはT，一致しない場合にはFを（　）内に記入しなさい。

1. （　） A study by a medical school researcher shows that any exercise could keep a brain young.
2. （　） We have available medications for treating Alzheimer's these days due to new findings.
3. （　） The study showed that people exercise improved their cognitive abilities.
4. （　） Researchers indicated that exercise lowers the risk of worsening memory problem.

B 音声を聴いて，次の英文の（　）内に適語を記入しなさい。　track 07

1. If you want to succeed, (　　) (　　) it.
2. The climate in this country is mild (　　) (　　) Malaysia.
3. She (　　) (　　) getting married with him.
4. I would like to (　　) (　　) (　　) the math class.

C 和文に合うように，（　）内の語句を並べかえて英文をつくりなさい。

1. 彼女は体の健康を維持するために定期的にピラティスをしている。
   (her, does, to, fit, she, Pilates, keep, regularly, body).

2. いったん何かをはじめたら，続けなければならない。
   (it, must, you, continue, begin, you, once, something).

3. 知恵は小出しにせよ（一度に使うな）。
   (use, a, you, your, a little, should, time, wisdom, at).

4. やる気がある限り，私は英語の勉強を続けるつもりです。
   (will, studying, as, I, as, last, can, long, continue, English, my motivation).

D 次の英語に相当する日本語を下から選び，記号で答えなさい。

1. dementia ( )
2. depression ( )
3. cognitive impairment ( )
4. delusion ( )
5. memory impairment ( )
6. aggression ( )
7. incontinence ( )
8. personality change ( )
9. senile ( )
10. wandering ( )

a. 老人(性) の　　b. うつ病　　c. 認知障害
d. 人格変化　　e. 記憶障害　　f. 徘徊
g. 認知症　　h. 失禁　　i. 攻撃性
j. 妄想

Unit 4 睡眠不足がもたらす健康被害

Are Sleep Problems a Growing Epidemic?

Voice of America, August 01, 2012

track 08

New research shows that a lack of sleep is a growing health problem around the world. Sleeplessness has been linked to such chronic illnesses as cardiovascular disease and diabetes.

Lack of sleep is not just a problem in developed nations. It's getting just as bad in developing countries as well.

Researchers at the University of Warwick Medical School in Coventry, England conducted the study. "Our purpose was to look at the existing data from eight different countries from both Africa and Asia. We came to estimate the prevalence of self-reported sleep problems across eight different populations. And also we tried to examine potential correlates of sleep problems in these populations," said lead author Dr. Saverio Stranges.

The research was conducted in Ghana, Tanzania, South Africa, India, Bangladesh, Vietnam, Indonesia and an urban area of Kenya. The study estimates 150 million adults in developing countries are suffering from sleep-related problems.

"There is biological evidence supporting the notion that sleep deprivation,

Notes:
epidemic／流行病　be linked to 〜／〜と関連がある　such A as B／BのようなA　chronic／慢性の　cardiovascular／心(臓)血管系の　diabetes／糖尿病　developed nation／先進国　developing country／発展途上国　〜 as well／〜もまた，そのうえ〜も　researcher／研究者　the University of Warwick Medical School／ウォーリック大学(英国ウェストミッドランズ州コヴェントリー市にある総合大学)医学部　both A and B／AもBも　come to 〜／〜するようになる　estimate／推定する，判断する　prevalence／流行　self-reported／自己報告の　population／住民　correlate／相互関係のあるもの　lead author／筆頭著者　urban area／都市部　suffer from 〜／〜に苦しむ　biological／生物学上の　notion／考え，見解　deprivation／不足

for example, may impair important physiological functions, including, for example, appetite or neuro-regenerative responses. And also have an impact on the immune system, which may actually explain the association of sleep with occurrence of many chronic diseases," he said.

He said sleep problems are also associated with unhealthy habits, such as smoking and a poor diet. Stranges says some people can actually sleep too much, such as the elderly, making them more prone to disease.

"In Western populations there is this common belief that a 24 hour society is driving these trends in sleep problems. The exposure to the Internet is likely an important contributor to this, if you like, epidemic of sleep problems in Western countries. Also, increasing prevalence of depression and anxiety disorders," Stranges said.

The study found that in developing countries depression and anxiety were also major factors in sleep problems. There was a higher prevalence among women than men.

Bangladesh, South Africa and Vietnam have extremely high levels of sleep problems.

"Sleep problems are becoming an important public health issue at least in some of these countries. And actually one interesting finding we had in this study was the striking variation of the prevalence of sleep problems across different populations. For example, we found that over 40 percent of people in Bangladesh may experience sleep problems, again with higher prevalence among women," he said.

On the other hand, India and Indonesia report relatively low levels of sleep

Notes:

impair／損なう　physiological／生理的　appetite／食欲　neuro-regenerative／神経再生の　have an impact on ～／～に影響を与える　immune system／免疫系　occurrence／発生　be associated with ～／～と関連している　A such as B／BのようなA　the elderly／高齢者　prone to ～／～の傾向がある　drive／駆り立てる　exposure／さらされること　contributor／一因　if you like／そう言いたければ　depression／うつ病　anxiety disorder／不安障害　public health／公衆衛生　issue／問題点　at least／少なくとも　striking／著しい　on the other hand／他方では

problems.

Stranges warned that sleeplessness could add to the already heavy disease burden in developing countries.

"Obviously, these are countries which are still facing the issue of infectious diseases and high mortality and morbidity from childhood-related diseases and maternal mortality. At the same time there is an increasing prevalence of chronic diseases in these populations," he said.

He said there are no simple solutions to sleep problems, which can be tied to the effects of poverty.

The study recommends that sleep patterns be included in assessing a population's overall health. It also says lifestyle changes should be considered before prescribing medication.

The study – Sleep problems: An Emerging Global Epidemic? – appears in the journal *Sleep*.

Notes:

add to ～／～を増す　burden／苦しみ, 重荷　face／直面する　infectious disease／感染症　mortality／死亡率　morbidity／罹患率　maternal／母の, 母性の　at the same time／同時に　be tied to ～／～に関係している　effect／影響　recommend／勧める　assess／評価する　overall／総体的な　prescribe／処方する　emerge／出現する, 浮かび上がる　*Sleep*／『スリープ』（睡眠を研究するSleep Research Societyが発行する学術雑誌）

Caffeine Found to Disrupt Internal Clock, Sleep Patterns

Voice of America, September 17, 2015

track 09

Researchers have discovered that caffeine can delay normal sleep times by as much as 40 minutes, if consumed three hours before anticipated bedtime.

The amount of caffeine associated with sleep disruption was equivalent to what is typically in two shots of espresso. Kenneth Wright, head of the Sleep and Chronobiology Laboratory at the University of Colorado in Boulder, said some coffee shop brews typically contain more caffeine than that.

Scientists have known for a long time that caffeine disrupts chemicals in the brain that affect wakefulness and blocks chemicals that promote sleep.

"This particular finding tells us that the timing of sleep and wakefulness will be pushed later because of an effect on the clock, not just promoting wakefulness chemicals in the brain," Wright said.

This is important because the natural process of circadian rhythm also affects hormone production and cell regeneration in the human body.

Not getting enough sleep can affect mood. It can also promote disorders like diabetes.

To look into caffeine's effect on the circadian clock, researchers at the

Notes:

disrupt／混乱させる　internal clock／体内時計　delay／遅らせる　as much as ～／～もの　consume／（たくさん）摂取する　anticipate／予想する　disruption／混乱, 中断　be equivalent to ～／～に相当する　the Sleep and Chronobiology Laboratory／睡眠・時間生物学研究所　the University of Colorado／コロラド大学（米国コロラド州ボルダーに本拠を置く州立大学）　brew／（1杯の）コーヒー　chemical／化学物質　affect／影響を与える　wakefulness／覚醒状態　promote／促進する　because of ～／～が原因で　circadian rhythm／概日リズム, 日周期リズム（生物に本来備わっている, 概ね一日を周期とするリズム）　regeneration／再生　disorder／疾患　circadian clock／概日時計

University of Colorado and the Medical Research Council Laboratory of Molecular Biology in Cambridge, England, first noted the sleep-wake cycles of five healthy volunteers.

Over the course of a 49-day study, investigators gave the participants 200 milligrams of caffeine, the equivalent amount found in two shots of espresso, a few hours before bed and noted how long it took them to fall asleep.

The volunteers were also exposed at night to bright light, which is known to disrupt sleep.

Caffeine did more than bright light in interrupting the circadian clock, and therefore patterns of sleep.

The researchers also looked at the biological function of a sleep hormone and found caffeine interrupted a core component of sleep at the cellular level.

Wright said adjusting one's biological clock in this way could also be beneficial.

"Another example of an implication of our findings is we may be able to use caffeine to help shift our clocks westward when we're traveling across many time zones," he said. "In this case, caffeine may help us adapt to jet lag much faster."

Notes:
the Medical Research Council Laboratory of Molecular Biology／MRC分子生物学研究所（医学や生物学に関連した基礎研究をおこなっている英国ケンブリッジにある国立研究所）　over the course of ～／～の間に　investigator／研究者　it takes A 時間 to ～／Aが～するのに時間がかかる　fall asleep／寝入る　be exposed to ～／～にさらされる　more than ～／～以上　interrupt／さえぎる，妨害する　component／構成要素　cellular／細胞の　adjust／調整する　beneficial／有益な　implication／それとなく示す意味　findings／（複数形で）研究結果　westward／西に向かって　time zone／タイムゾーン（時間帯：同じ標準時間を利用する地域・区分）　adapt to ～／～に順応する　jet lag／時差ぼけ

The findings, published in the journal *Science Translational Medicine*, also suggest people who want to wake up earlier in the morning might consider giving up that nighttime cup of java.

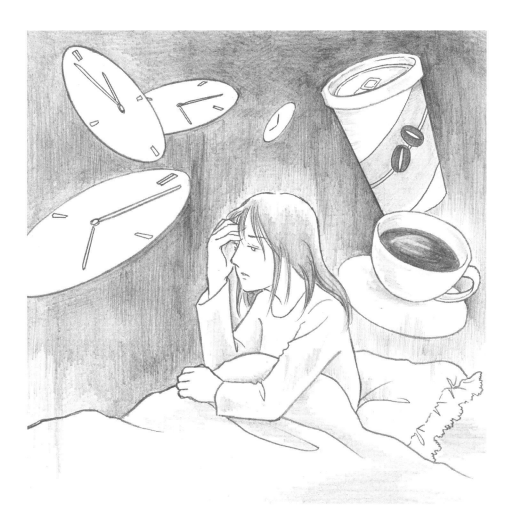

Notes:

Science Translational Medicine／『サイエンス・トランスレーショナル・メディシン』（米国科学振興協会によって発行されている学術雑誌で，『サイエンス』の姉妹誌）　give up 〜／〜をやめる　java／《米俗》コーヒー

練習問題

A 本文の内容に合うように，各英文の（　）内に入るもっとも適当な語句をそれぞれ1つずつ選びなさい。

1. Recently, lack of sleep is becoming a problem in (developed countries, developing countries, eight different countries).
2. We see that women suffer from sleep problem more than men in (South Africa, Indonesia, Bangladesh).
3. Sleep problems have a tie with (infectious diseases, maternal mortality, poverty).
4. The research shows that our circadian rhythm could be affected by (caffeine, chemicals, cell regeneration).

B 音声を聴いて，次の英文の（　）内に適語を記入しなさい。　　track 10

1. Smoking could (　　) (　　) (　　) lifestyle-related diseases.
2. The trip was canceled (　　) (　　) bad weather.
3. You can (　　) (　　) (　　) (　　) the public.
4. The chair (　　) (　　) (　　) the weather all the time.

C 和文に合うように，（　）内の語句を並べかえて英文をつくりなさい。

1. 彼は辛辣な意見を言う傾向がある。
   (make, prone, he, remarks, cutting, to, is).

2. 1マイルは約1.6キロメートルに相当する。
   (about, to, is, 1.6 kilometers, mile, equivalent, one).

3. ジャックが自転車を修理するのに3時間かかった。
   (Jack, to, bicycle, took, it, repair, hours, his, three).

4. フライドポテトのような脂っこい食べ物は私たちの健康に悪い。
   (are, foods, for, as, our health, French fries, fatty, such, bad).

D 次の英語に相当する日本語を下から選び，記号で答えなさい。
1. alcoholism　　　　　(　)　2. autonomic imbalance　(　)
3. cerebral infarction　(　)　4. delirium　　　　　　(　)
5. neurologist　　　　 (　)　6. drug abuse　　　　　(　)
7. insomnia　　　　　 (　)　8. maladjustment　　　 (　)
9. mania　　　　　　 (　)　10. neurosis　　　　　　(　)

a. 不眠症　　　　　　b. 神経症　　　　　　c. 不適応
d. 躁病　　　　　　　e. 神経科医　　　　　f. 脳梗塞
g. 薬物乱用　　　　　h. 譫妄（せんもう）　i. 自律神経失調症
j. アルコール依存症

Unit 5 喫煙に安全なレベルは存在するのか?

Study: There's No Safe Level of Smoking

Voice of America, December 06, 2016

track 11

There is no safe level of smoking, according to a new study. (1)[day, your life, shorten, one cigarette, even, a, can], while quitting later in life can add years.

We all know smoking cigarettes is harmful. But some people think if they only have one cigarette per day, or 10 or fewer, they are in the clear for smoking-related diseases including lung cancer and heart disease.

Not so fast, say researchers at the U.S. National Cancer Institute. The investigators conducted the first study looking at the health impact of so-called low-intensity smoking.

Dr. Maki Inoue-Choi, an epidemiologist at NCI, led the study.

The results were based on questionnaires filled out by smokers taking part in a large, long-term study of more than 290,000 adults being conducted by the National Institutes of Health.

"In our study, we found the kind of smokers who consistently smoke less than one cigarette per day over their lifetime were 1.6 times more likely to die during the study compared to never-smokers. And (2)adults who consistently smoked between one and ten cigarettes per day were 1.9 times more likely to die during the study than never-smokers," said Inoue-Choi.

The health risks were lower among former low-intensity smokers compared to those who continued to puff away, and the risk of serious illness dropped the earlier someone quits.

The results of the research were published in *JAMA Internal Medicine*.

The study, part of NIH's large prospective AARP Diet and Health study, includes adults from 59 to 82. Questionnaires were sent to participants in 2004-2005. Some of the smokers began at age 15 or younger.

During follow-up 10 years later, (3)investigators found smokers who puffed one cigarette or less per day increased their risk of lung cancer by nine percent compared to never-smokers. And lung cancer death was 12 times higher among those (4   ) indulged in one to 10 cigarettes per day.

There were also increases in early death from other causes. People who smoked between one and 10 cigarettes a day had more than six times the risk of dying from respiratory diseases, like emphysema, than never-smokers and about one and half times the risk of succumbing to cardiovascular disease.

Numerous negative health effects of smoking have been researched and described over the years, beginning with the U.S. Surgeon General's report in 1964. But (5)the study in the *JAMA journal* is the first to actually look at the health impacts of low cigarette consumption.

Another study involving some 170,000 participants, published recently in *the American Journal of Preventive Medicine*, also found it's never too late (6   ) quit. The participants were also in the AARP Diet and Health study.

Even among those who stopped smoking in their 60's, they were 23 percent less likely (7   ) die early compared to those who kept smoking in their 70s, according to lead researcher Sarah Nash.

Norman Edelman is a pulmonologist and a senior medical consultant to the American Lung Association.

Edelman said both studies were extremely well done and their findings convincing because of their enormous size.

50　Edelman said he has a large number (　8　) patients who say they can't quit.

"And you know I can now pull out data from the study we were talking about and say, "No, no, no (9)you can actually prolong your life even if you're well into your 60s and quit."

55　Edelman said the studies show (10)it is never too early and never too late to kick the habit.

Notes:

according to 〜／〜によれば　quit／やめる　in the clear／安全で, 危険を脱して　lung／肺　cancer／がん　Not so fast.／そんなに急ぐな。早合点するな。　the U. S. National Cancer Institute／米国国立がん研究所（略称はNCI）　investigator／研究者　look at 〜／〜を検討する　low-intensity／軽度の　epidemiologist／疫学者　be based on 〜／〜に基づいている　questionnaire／アンケート　fill out 〜／〜に記入する　take part in 〜／〜に参加する　more than 〜／〜より多い　the National Institutes of Health／米国国立衛生研究所（略称はNIH）　consistently／持続的に, 絶えず　less than 〜／〜より少ない　compared to 〜／〜と比べると　between A and B／AからBまでの間　puff away／（たばこを）ふかす　the earlier someone quit／（人が）やめるのが早ければ早いほど　JAMA Internal Medicine／『JAMAインターナル・メディシン』（米国医師会雑誌JAMAの内科版）　prospective／期待される　AARP Diet and Health study／米国退職者協会（American Association of Retired Persons）食事・健康調査　participant／参加者, 関係者　follow-up／追跡調査　indulge in 〜／〜にふける, 〜を楽しむ　respiratory／呼吸器の　emphysema／肺気腫　succumb to 〜／〜に屈する　cardiovascular／心（臓）血管の　numerous／非常に多くの　begin with 〜／〜で始まる　surgeon general／《米》公衆衛生局長官　consumption／消費（量）　the American Journal of Preventive Medicine／『アメリカン・ジャーナル・オブ・プリベンティブ・メディシン』　keep 〜ing／〜し続ける　pulmonologist／呼吸器専門医　senior medical consultant／シニア医療コンサルタント　the American Lung Association／米国肺協会　extremely／きわめて　findings／（複数形で）研究結果　convincing／説得力のある　because of 〜／〜の理由で　enormous／非常に大きい　prolong／延ばす　even if 〜／たとえ〜だとしても　kick the habit／習慣をやめる, 悪習を絶つ

練習問題

A 本文中の (4) (6) (7) (8) に適語を入れなさい（音声を参考にしてもよい）。

　　(4) (　　　)　(6) (　　　　)　(7) (　　　　)　(8) (　　　　　)

B (1) が「一日一本のたばこでも命を縮めることがある」という意味になるように [　　　] 内の語句を並べかえなさい（音声を参考にしてもよい）。

C 下線部 (2) (3) (5) (9) (10) を日本語に直しなさい。

(2)

(3)

(5)

(9)

(10)

D 次の説明に合う語を英文中から選びなさい。

(11) a very serious disease in which cells in the body grow in an uncontrolled way (　　　　)
(12) the possibility that something bad may happen (　　　　)
(13) something without which something else would not happen (　　　　)
(14) the act or process of using up something (　　　　)
(15) a person who is receiving medical care (　　　　)

Review (Unit 1〜Unit 4)

A 英文の (　) 内に入る語を次ページ上から選んで記入し，英文を日本語に直しなさい。

1. He applied to Harvard University, but failed (　) get accepted. (Unit 1)

2. I go (　) a walk every morning. (Unit 2)

3. Mary pointed (　) the need for better training. (Unit 3)

4. I gave (　　) alcohol while I was pregnant. (Unit 4)

> up,　　for,　　to,　　out

B 和文に合うように，(　　)内の語句を並べかえて英文をつくりなさい。

1. 人生はしばしば航海にたとえられる。(Unit 1)
   (to, is, a voyage, likened, life, often).

2. 私の意見では，あなたは重大な間違いをしている。(Unit 2)
   (making, opinion, mistake, you're, my, serious, in, a).

3. 寒すぎてコートなしでは外出できない。(Unit 3)
   (is, out, a coat, to, cold, go, too, it, without).

4. （一方でとても便利であるが）他方で，車はとんでもない量の汚染を引き起こす。(Unit 4)
   (hand, the, pollution, other, a huge amount of, cause, cars, on).

C 次の英語に相当する日本語を下から選び，記号で答えなさい。

1. infant　　　　　　(　) 　2. mortality　　　　　(　)
3. consumer　　　　 (　) 　4. cardiologist　　　　(　)
5. arthritis　　　　　(　) 　6. symptom　　　　　(　)
7. artery　　　　　　(　) 　8. deprivation　　　　(　)
9. anxiety　　　　　 (　) 　10. disruption　　　　(　)

> a. 不足　　　　　　　b. 消費者　　　　　　　c. 混乱
> d. 動脈　　　　　　　e. 幼児　　　　　　　　f. 不安
> g. 死亡率　　　　　　h. 循環器専門医　　　　i. 症状
> j. 関節炎

Unit 6 アフリカの発展途上国における子宮頸がん対策

Cancer a Public Health Concern in Africa's Developing Countries

Voice of America, November 12, 2014

track 12

YAOUNDÉ — Medical experts say cervical cancer continues to be the leading cause of cancer-related deaths in Sub-Saharan Africa. A majority die of ignorance. Less than one percent of women are scanned for the disease. Free vaccination campaigns for 9 to 13 years old girls are ongoing.

Medical doctors from Chad, Gabon, Republic of Congo, Equatorial Guinea, Cameroon and the Central African Republic say the impact of chronic diseases such as cancer is steadily growing in many low- and middle-income countries. Dr. Ndikum Donald, a cancer expert working in the Chadian capital, N'Djamena, said early detection is essential to improving chances for recovery.

"Low income countries are the most affected simply because in the developed countries they have an organized program, regular programs where they screen women every three to five years. So in countries where the screening programs are developed, the cancer is well controlled," said Donald.

Notes:

public health／公衆衛生　developing country／発展途上国　Yaoundé／ヤウンデ（カメルーンの首都）　cervical cancer／子宮頸がん　Sub-Saharan Africa／サハラ砂漠以南のアフリカ　die of ～／～が原因で死ぬ　ignorance／無知, 無学　less then ～／～より少ない　scan／入念に調べる　vaccination／ワクチンの予防接種　ongoing／継続中の　Chad／チャド（北アフリカ中央部の共和国）　Gabon／ガボン（アフリカ南西部の共和国）　Republic of Congo／コンゴ共和国（アフリカ中部の国）　Equatorial Guinea／赤道ギニア（アフリカ中西部の共和国）　Cameroon／カメルーン（アフリカ西部の共和国）　the Central African Republic／中央アフリカ共和国　chronic／慢性の　A such as B／BのようなA　steadily／着実に, 絶え間なく　low- and middle-income／低・中所得の　Chadian／チャドの　N'Djamena／ンジャメナ（チャドの首都）　detection／発見, 探知　be essential to ～／～にとって必要不可欠である　affected／影響を受けた,（病気に）冒された　simply because ～／～という理由だけで　developed country／先進国　organized／きちんとした, 準備周到な　screen／検査する　screening／検査

Professor Anderson Doh of Cameroon's cancer committee said in his country alone they have been detecting 14,000 cases of cancer each year, and 4,000 are cancers of the cervix. He said most are reported in middle-aged women and the patients suffer longer and die sooner than those in high-income countries.

"The numbers are increasing partly because the population is increasing in number, but also the lifestyle that is changing is contributing to this. Take smoking for instance. If you take cancer of the cervix, cancer of the breast even cancer of the prostate now, we find even some young men who came to ask for help at an early age," said Doh.

Professor Doh said governments in Sub-Saharan countries should act quickly. He said all women, regardless of economic status or geographic location, should have access to accurate, affordable cervical cancer screenings. He urged people to live healthier lives as a means of preventing the disease.

"We have solutions to them. Prevention, primary prevention by avoiding smoking, eating roughly. A square meal should have vegetables once in a while, fruits and all that. Obesity is a problem and this obesity predisposes us to certain cancers," advised Doh.

Cancer of the cervix is the leading cause of cancer-related death for women in the countries which have organized screening for girl children from 9 to 13 years old. Doh said the campaign is free.

"The vaccine is free. There are two types of vaccines in the market.

Notes:
committee／委員会　～ alone／ただ～だけ，～のみ　detect／見つけ出す　cervix／子宮頸部　suffer／苦しむ　high-income／高所得の　partly because ～／ひとつには～の理由で　in number／数の上で　contribute to ～／～の一因となる　take ～ for instance／～を例にとる　prostate／前立腺　regardless of ～／～に関係なく　geographic／地理的な　have access to ～／～を利用できる，～が手に入る　accurate／正確な　affordable／手ごろな価格の　urge A to ～／Aに～するように促す　live a healthy life／健康的な生活を送る　as a means of ～／～の手段として　prevent／予防する　solution／解決策　prevention／予防　square meal／まともな食事　once in a while／ときどき　and all that／その他もろもろ　obesity／（病的な）肥満　predispose A to B／AをBに罹りやすくする　vaccine／ワクチン

Gardasil and Cervarix. We chose Gardasil as our first," said Doh.

40　Health experts say cervical cancer is preventable, but each year approximately 80 percent of cancer-related deaths occur in developing countries, where less than one percent of women have been screened for the disease.

Notes:

Gardasil／ガーダシル（米国製の子宮頸がん予防ワクチン）　Cervarix／サーバリックス（米国製の子宮頸がん予防ワクチン）　preventable／予防可能な　approximately／およそ

WHO Stresses Value of Vaccine in Preventing Cervical Cancer

Voice of America, December 02, 2014

track 13

GENEVA — Cervical cancer, a preventable sexually transmitted disease, kills an estimated 270,000 women each year, 85 percent of whom live in developing countries, the World Health Organization said.

More than a half million women each year become infected with the human papillomavirus, which causes cervical cancer, the U.N. agency said.

Marleen Temmerman, director of the WHO Department of Reproductive Health and Research, said that a safe, effective vaccine exists to stop the infection and that it's advisable for girls age 9 to 13 to get vaccinated before they become sexually active. The vaccine provides immunity for at least 10 years, and no booster shot is recommended.

"New studies have shown that, traditionally, we used to give three injections to the girls to immunize them fully," she said. "But we have shown now that two is enough, which is a major kind of step in the right direction because it reduces the number of injections and the cost."

The cost of one HPV injection can be as high as $140, a price out of reach for most people in developing countries.

The World Health Organization said girls in more than 55 countries are protected by routine administration of HPV vaccine, and a growing number

Notes:

WHO／世界保健機関（the World Health Organization）　Geneva／ジュネーブ（スイス南西部の都市，WHOの本部がある）　sexually transmitted disease／性感染症　estimated／およそ　more than ～／～より多い　become infected with ～／～に感染する　human papillomavirus／（子宮頸がんの原因となる）ヒト乳頭腫ウイルス，ヒトパピローマウイルス（略語はHPV）　the U. N. agency／国連（United Nations）機関　Department of Reproductive Health and Research／リプロダクティブ・ヘルスと研究部門　infection／感染症，伝染病　advisable／勧められる，賢明な　vaccinate／ワクチン注射をする　immunity／免疫（性）　at least／少なくとも　booster shot／追加接種　recommend／勧める　used to ～／以前は～したものだ　injection／注射　immunize／免疫性を与える　the number of ～／～の数　out of reach／手の届かない，力の及ばない　administration／投与　a growing number of ～／ますます多くの～

of countries are providing vaccine with support from the GAVI Alliance, a public-private global health partnership.

More methods are now available to screen women to identify pre-cancerous lesions. According to new guidelines, a woman whose screening proves negative needs only to be rescreened within 10 years, which represents a major cost savings for health systems.

The U.N. health agency said that more than 1 million women worldwide are living with cervical cancer, many with no access to curative treatment or palliative care. Temmerman attributed much of this situation to cost issues and to the low priority that many health systems place on dealing with this issue. But she said countries in eastern and southern Africa are developing national cancer survival plans.

"It is still at the pilot phase," she said, "so they do demonstration projects to show that HPV vaccination is feasible. Secondly, they do the testing. So they start with women who go to family planning, women who go to the health sector for other reasons. And in some of the countries, like in Kenya, they now do mobile clinic outreach."

The objectives are to spread the message that cervical cancer is dangerous and preventable and to stress the importance of screening and treatment if cervical cancer is discovered.

Notes:

with support from 〜／〜の支援によって　the GAVI Alliance／ワクチンと予防接種のための世界同盟（旧称は Global Alliance for Vaccines and Immunization）　public-private／官民の　partnership／協力　identify／明らかにする, 確認する　pre-cancerous／前がん性の　lesion／病変　according to 〜／〜に従って　prove／判明する　rescreen／再検査する　represent／意味する, 表す　saving／節約　live with 〜／〜を受け入れる, 〜を我慢する　with no access to 〜／〜が利用不可能で　curative／病気に効く　treatment／治療　palliative care／緩和ケア　attribute A to B／AをBに帰する, AをBのせいにする　place low priority on 〜／〜の重要性が低いとみなす　deal with 〜／〜に対処する, 〜に取り組む　pilot phase／試験段階　demonstration project／実証プロジェクト　feasible／実行できる, 実現可能な　start with 〜／〜から始める　family planning／（受胎調節による）家族計画　health sector／保健・医療部門（具体的には, 病院やクリニックなどを指す）　mobile clinic outreach／移動式クリニックサービス　objective／目標, 目的

練習問題

A 本文の内容に合うように，各英文の（　）内に入るもっとも適当な語句をそれぞれ1つずつ選びなさい。

1. Medical doctors say the impact of (acute, chronic, congenital) diseases is steadily growing in many low-income countries.
2. The professor says the patients in Cameroon suffer longer and die sooner than those in (high-income, low-income, middle-income) countries.
3. More than a half million women each year become infected with (HCV, HIV, HPV), which causes cervical cancer.
4. More than 1 million women with cervical cancer are living with no access to curative treatment or (intensive, palliative, terminal) care.

B 音声を聴いて，次の英文の（　）内に適語を記入しなさい。　track 14

1. The actress (　　) (　　) a heart attack.
2. We like to order Mexican food (　　) (　　) (　　) (　　).
3. It'll cost (　　) (　　) 800 dollars.
4. The policeman kicked the knife (　　) (　　) (　　).

C 和文に合うように，（　）内の語句を並べかえて英文をつくりなさい。

1. 病院職員数は15パーセント削減されるだろう。
   (in, 15％, decreased, be, hospital staff, by, will, number).

2. 彼女は両親の考えに関係なく家を出るつもりだ。
   (think, of, is, her parents, leave home, what, to, regardless, going, she).

3. ますます多くの人が赤身の肉の摂取量を減らしたがっている。
   (choosing, people, growing, of, red meat, a, to eat, number, less, are).

4. メアリーは，自分が成功したのは猛勉強して少し運がよかったからだと考えている。
   (luck, her success, and, work, to, Mary, a little, attributes, hard).

Unit 6

D 次の英語に相当する日本語を下から選び，記号で答えなさい。

1. cervical cancer （　）　2. breast cancer （　）
3. gastric cancer （　）　4. ovarian cancer （　）
5. lung cancer （　）　6. esophageal cancer （　）
7. pancreatic cancer （　）　8. prostate cancer （　）
9. colon cancer （　）　10. liver cancer （　）

a. 膵臓がん　　　b. 肝臓がん　　　c. 食道がん
d. 胃がん　　　　e. 前立腺がん　　f. 結腸(大腸)がん
g. 乳がん　　　　h. 子宮頸がん　　i. 卵巣がん
j. 肺がん

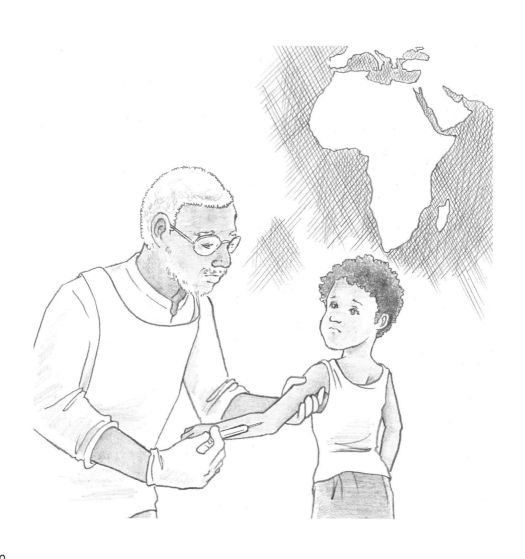

Unit 7 脊髄損傷の痛みを和らげる新しい手術

New Surgical Techniques Help Relieve Pain from Spinal Injury

Voice of America, October 28, 2016

🔊 track 15

DENVER — Being in a wheelchair has never slowed Jon Forbes down. But for 14 years after his spinal cord injury, Forbes says something else nearly broke his will to live. It was pain - electric shocks of pain - in areas of his body that were paralyzed. "It was horrible, excruciating, and it never stopped," he recalled. "You wake up, it's there. All day, it's there. You go to bed, it's there."

According to the World Health Organization, roughly 25 million people around the world live with a spinal cord injury. The injuries are well-known for causing paralysis and difficulty with using legs and hands. Less recognized is the common side effect Forbes described -- neuropathic pain, which creates feelings of electric shocks and stabs in parts of the body that no longer have regular sensation. In roughly 10 percent of cases, this neuropathic pain can be so relentless, that victims consider suicide. Forbes did consider suicide.

"I had tried pretty much every kind of drug, tried exercise, tried you name it. Anything and everything to try and get this pain to stop. And it wouldn't.

Notes:
relieve／緩和する　spinal injury／脊髄の損傷　Denver／デンバー（米国コロラド州の州都）　slow ~ down／~を不活発にさせる　spinal cord injury／脊髄損傷　will／意志　electric shock／電気ショック, 電撃　paralyze／麻痺させる　horrible／ひどい　excruciating／極度に痛い　recall／回想する　according to ~／~によれば　the World Health Organization／世界保健機関　roughly／おおよそ　live with ~／~を受け入れる, ~に耐える　be well-known for ~／~でよく知られている　paralysis／麻痺　side effect／副作用　neuropathic／神経障害性の　stab／刺すような痛み　no longer ~／もはや~でない　sensation／感覚　relentless／絶え間なく続く　victim／被害者, 罹病者　suicide／自殺　pretty much／ほとんど　you name it／そのほか何でも　try and get A to ~／努力してAを~させる

And I was working at an investment bank and decided this was it." He starts to tear up as he remembers that time of his life. "I quit my job, and decided, this was going to be the end. I just couldn't take it."

But then, he learned about a Denver neurosurgeon who uses spinal surgery to stop so-called "suicidal pain."

The last resort

Scott Falci acknowledges, "Patients, when they ultimately come to me, I'm kind of a last resort." As the chief neurosurgical consultant at Denver's Craig Hospital, which specializes in spinal cord injury rehabilitation, Falci has helped hundreds of paralyzed patients who suffer excruciating neuropathic pain.

"You could cut them with a knife, they wouldn't feel it. You could put a blow torch on their foot. I'm being extreme here. They wouldn't feel it," he stresses. "Yet they'll tell me, 'my foot is on fire, as if someone has set it on fire.' 'Battery acid's on my foot', and they can be very site specific. They'll say, 'I have electricity running from my hip to my knee,' or 'the bottom of my foot, it's on fire.' 'At the ankles it's somebody stabbing me with a knife.' They feel the pain precisely in very specific areas, but if you were to touch them on those areas, they couldn't tell you."

For spinal cord patients, conventional pain therapies frequently fail, so often doctors suggest the pain is "in their head." But, Falci says, it's actually in their spinal cord. He resolves it with surgery.

Notes:

investment bank／投資銀行　this was it／これで最後だ　tear up／目に涙をためる　take it／我慢する　neurosurgeon／神経外科医　so-called／いわゆる　"suicidal pain"／「自殺したい衝動に駆られる痛み」　last resort／最後の手段　acknowledge／認める　ultimately／最終的に　kind of 〜／ある意味では〜　the chief neurosurgical consultant／神経外科の主任　Craig Hospital／クレイグ病院（米国コロラド州デンバーにある世界的に有名なリハビリ専門病院）　specialize in 〜／〜を専門にしている　rehabilitation／リハビリテーション　hundreds of 〜／何百もの〜　blow torch／ガスバーナー　extreme／極端な　stress／強調する　be on fire／燃えている　as if 〜／まるで〜であるかのように　set 〜 on fire／〜に火をつける　battery acid／蓄電池で使用される希硫酸　site specific／部位特異的な　electricity／電気　hip／尻, 腰　knee／膝　bottom／（足の）裏　ankle／足首　stab／突き刺す　precisely／正確に　be to touch／触ってみようとする　conventional／従来の　therapy／治療　frequently／しばしば　resolve／解決する　surgery／外科手術

Revolution in the OR

40 Under lamps as bright as the sun, half a dozen surgical assistants help Falci for hours, just to reveal the spinal cord. He explains, "You have to open up the skin, the muscles, you have to get to the skeleton, and you have to remove some bone in the back of the skeleton to even get to see the spinal cord."

45 Finally, the spinal cord is revealed, glistening, white, alive. Falci seeks out pearl-colored "root entry zones," each the size of a small button, filled with thousands of cells. These are where nerve bundles bring sensations from the body and root into the spinal cord. "These nerve cells that come from different parts of the body don't travel all the way up to the brain," he 50 notes. "They connect first with other nerve cells in the spinal cord which lets them communicate signals to the brain."

Using a pin-sized electrode, Falci carefully probes two millimeters into these areas, to touch relay nerves in the spinal cord that speed sensory information toward the brain. Mostly he gets a calm electric signal. Then, 55 there's a spike, the sign of hyperactive nerve cells. Falci calls them "hot spots" — seizure-like areas of the nerve cells firing with high energy when they shouldn't be firing.

He says hot spots can trigger suicidal pain. "So you can imagine, the hyperactive areas of the spinal cord, almost every second of their life, 60 bombarding their brain and telling them they're with pain."

Notes:

revolution／革命　OR／手術室 (operation room)　lamp／照明器具　surgical assistant／手術助手　reveal／見せる, あらわにする　open up ～／～を切開する　muscle／筋肉　skeleton／骨格　remove／取り除く　glistening／ギラギラ光っている　seek out ～／～を探し出す　"root entry zone"／「神経根進入部」　filled with ～／～でいっぱいの　thousands of ～／何千もの～　nerve bundles／神経束　root into ～／～の中に(根のように)入り込む　all the way up to ～／～までずっと　pin-sized electrode／ピンほどの大きさの電極　probe／探る　relay nerves／介在神経 (interneuron)　spike／棘波, (神経の)活動電位　hyperactive／機能が亢進している　seizure-like／発作のような　fire／(神経が)興奮する　trigger／誘発する　almost every second of one's life／人生のほぼすべての間　bombard／攻める

Using heat, Falci kills each hot spot. There can be hundreds, so meticulously, he moves up the spinal column, killing hot spots.

He also does something that neurosurgeons have considered out of the question. "We didn't believe the spinal cord below the level of injury could possibly send signals to the brain," he explains, but even if an injury has completely cut the spinal cord in half, Falci finds and kills hot spots below the injury.

He explains that nerve signals coming in from the body can detour around a spinal cord injury. He likens this to how highway drivers detour onto local lanes to avoid an accident, then after the accident, they merge back on the highway. When it's hyperactive nerve signals creating a detour in the body, Falci says they carry false pain signals. So by killing hot spots below the injury, he eliminates more pain. "Eighty-five percent of the time, we can get rid of sharps, burns, electricals, and stabs."

New lease on life

Falci says this can be life changing. It was for Jon Forbes, who got this surgery two years ago, and reports, "I'm a pretty happy person these days." Just two months after the operation, Forbes landed a new job — as the deputy treasurer for the state of Colorado. "I'm not 100％ without pain," he admits, "but I can live, and I want to live, which is . . . thank God for saving my life, Dr. Falci."

Falci plans to publish new research that maps this "detouring" nervous system. His work makes him confident that there's more to discover about how the human body deals with injury and pain.

Notes:

meticulously／注意深く　spinal column／脊柱　out of the question／問題にならない，不可能な　even if ～／たとえ～だとしても　in half／半分に　detour／回り道をする，回り道　liken A to B／AをBに例える　local lane／一般道　merge／合流する　false／誤った　eliminate／除去する　get rid of ～／～を取り除く　sharp／鋭い痛み　burn／焼け付くような痛み　electrical／電気を受けたような痛み　new lease on life／元気を取り戻すこと　these days／最近　land a job／職を得る　deputy treasurer／会計担当補佐　thank God for ～／～を神に感謝する　publish／（論文を）発表する　map／解読する　deal with ～／～に対処する

練習問題

A 次の英文が本文の内容に一致する場合にはT，一致しない場合にはFを（　）内に記入しなさい。

1. (　) It was not being in a wheelchair but the pain Jon Forbes had in his paralyzed areas which almost broke his will to live.
2. (　) According to WHO, more than thirty million people around the world live with a spinal cord injury.
3. (　) Scott Falci is a neurosurgeon at Denver's Craig Hospital and he has helped hundreds of patients who suffer severe neuropathic pain by rehabilitating their injured knees.
4. (　) Having undergone a spinal surgery at Denver's Craig Hospital, Jon Forbes found his pains were much relieved and he could take on a new job.

B 音声を聴いて，次の英文の（　）内に適語を記入しなさい。　track 16

1. The product license is (　　) (　　) available.
2. Jane (　　) (　　) (　　) grief at the news of her sister's death.
3. I have to go to see a doctor as I can't (　　) (　　) (　　) my cough.
4. Mr. Smith is hard to (　　) (　　).

C 和文に合うように，（　）内の語句を並べかえて英文をつくりなさい。

1. グリーン博士は腫瘍免疫学における研究でよく知られています。
   (his, in, well-known, tumor immunology, for, is, Dr. Greene, research).

2. その守衛は私たちを建物の中にどうしても入れてくれなかった。
   (the, us, let, guard, security, the building, wouldn't, into).

3. その患者はまるで一週間眠っていないように見えた。
   (hadn't, the patient, a week, if, he, looked, slept, for, as).

4. この小道を行くと丘の頂上まで行けますよ。
   (the hill, this path, take, all, you, the, will, way, to, of, the top).

D 次の英語に相当する日本語を下から選び、記号で答えなさい。

1. surgery　　　　　　　（　）　2. neurosurgeon　　　　　（　）
3. surgical assistant　　（　）　4. transfusion　　　　　　（　）
5. resuscitation　　　　（　）　6. emergency room　　　（　）
7. anesthesia　　　　　（　）　8. amputation　　　　　　（　）
9. paralysis　　　　　　（　）　10. artificial respiration　（　）

　　a. 輸血　　　　　b. 切断　　　　　c. 手術助手
　　d. 人工呼吸　　　e. 蘇生　　　　　f. 緊急救命室
　　g. 外科手術　　　h. 麻痺　　　　　i. 神経外科医
　　j. 麻酔

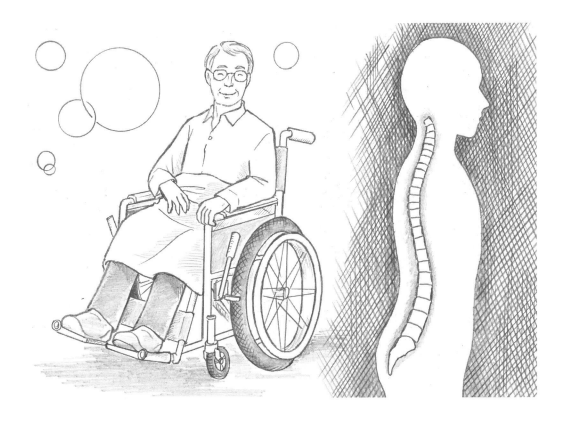

Unit 8 有害化学物質の行き着く先

Climate Change Could Increase Oceanic Mercury

Voice of America, January 27, 2017

🔊 track 17

Climate change is never as simple as 'the world is getting warmer'; it is a complicated string of cause and effect.

And a new study suggests one of those strings could have a huge impact on some of the seafood we eat.

5 **Extreme weather, extreme runoff**

The new research is a collaboration between researchers at Umeå University and the Swedish University of Agricultural Sciences, and is being published today in the journal *Science Advances*.

It points to a link between extreme weather, increased water runoff and
10 potentially massive increases in the levels of dangerous mercury in "coastal zones, coastal seas and lakes"—any area, lead author Erik Björn told VOA "which receives large input from runoff."

The study comes to its conclusions based on evidence that predicts that

---

Notes:

oceanic／大洋の　mercury／水銀　never as ～ as A／Aほど決して～ではない　complicated／複雑な　a string of ～／～の連鎖　cause and effect／原因と結果　have a huge impact on ～／～に莫大な影響を及ぼす　extreme weather／異常気象　runoff／（地中に吸収されずに地表を流れる）表面流水　collaboration／共同研究　Umeå University／ウメオ大学（スウェーデンのウメオにある公立大学）　the Swedish University of Agricultural Sciences／スウェーデン農業科学大学　journal／専門誌　*Science Advances*／『サイエンス・アドバンシーズ』（米国科学振興協会〔AAAS〕が刊行する学際的なオープンアクセスの電子版専門誌）　point to ～／～を指摘する　a link between A and B／AとBの間のつながり, 関係　a massive increase in ～／～の大幅な増加　"coastal zones, coastal seas and lakes"／「沿岸域, 近海および湖」　lead author／筆頭著者　input／流入　come to one's conclusions／独自の結論を出す　predict／予測する

"global warming is expected to increase runoff and input of organic matter to aquatic ecosystems in large regions of the Northern hemisphere..."

That 15 to 30 percent increase in water runoff of farms and lawns and roads, the study says, will cloud ocean water, resulting in "reductions in the production of phytoplankton via photosynthesis." Phytoplanktons serve as the primary bottom rung of the food chain throughout the world's oceans and lakes.

With less sunlight and a lot of organic material, the environment begins to favor bacteria called zooplankton which feed on all the junk washed into the water.

That's bad for two reasons: the first is that the runoff carries "a greater discharge of mercury and organic carbon to coastal ecosystems, which leads to higher levels of mercury in the small animals living there." The study estimates the amount of mercury in zooplankton could jump "by 200 to 700 percent."

Second, all that runoff means animals that were eating primarily phytoplankton have to eat more zooplankton, and that means even more mercury gets into their systems, and up and up through the food chain.

From the water to the dinner table

It is hard to overestimate the negative effects that mercury has on humans, especially children. Speaking with VOA, Björn laid out just how dangerous

Notes:
organic matter／有機物　aquatic ecosystem／水界生態系　the Northern hemisphere／北半球　water runoff of 〜／〜からの表面流水　cloud／濁らせる　ocean water／海水　result in 〜／〜の結果になる　reduction in 〜／〜の減少　phytoplankton／植物プランクトン　via 〜／〜を通して　photosynthesis／光合成　serve as 〜／〜の役割を果たす　bottom rung／底辺, 一番下の段　food chain／食物連鎖　favor／に有利である, 好都合である　zooplankton／動物プランクトン　feed on 〜／〜を餌にする　junk／くず　discharge／流出量　organic carbon／有機炭素　coastal ecosystem／沿岸生態系　lead to 〜／〜をもたらす, 〜につながる　estimate／推定する, 見積もる　primarily／主として　one's system／（人・動物の）体　it is hard to overestimate 〜／〜は計り知れない　have a negative effect on 〜／〜に悪影響を及ぼす　speak with 〜／〜と話す　lay out 〜／〜を明確に説明する

the chemical is: "Mercury is considered one of the top ten chemicals of public health concern by the World Health Organization."

In the European Union, he notes, "1.8 million children are born each year with prenatal exposure levels of methylmercury considered unsafe." And the adverse effects of mercury poisoning in the EU are "estimated to [cost] 90 million Euro per year."

Those numbers are current, he says, and if climate change leads to increased erosion, the health effects will get worse and the associated price tag, higher.

One quick note, the climate change model the team used assumes we keep pumping carbon into the atmosphere at the same rate we do today. If we cut back on emissions, it could lower the amount of mercury that ends up on our dinner table.

Björn also pointed to global efforts like the 2013 Minamata Convention on Mercury, signed by 128 countries and ratified by 36 with a sense of optimism. It deeply restricts mercury mining, its use and its disposal. "We have great hope" he said, that if the convention takes hold, "that the exposure of mercury to ecosystems and humans will decrease in the future."

The link between climate change, erosion and ultimately more mercury in our systems is long, involved and complicated, just like the climate. But by following the mercury, these researchers present a fascinating cautionary tale of how seemingly unrelated events can lead to unexpected, unintended and dangerous outcomes.

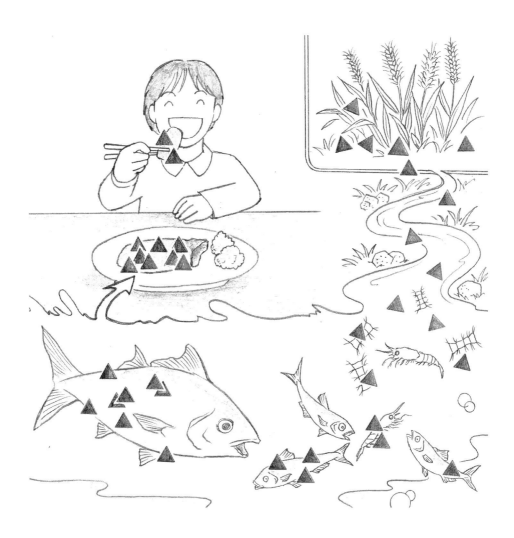

Notes:
seemingly／表面的には，一見　outcome／結果

Fast Food Packaging Could Be Dangerous

Voice of America, February 02, 2017

🔊 track 18

Fast food packaging contains chemicals that could be harmful, a new study suggests.

Writing in the journal *Environmental Science & Technology Letters*, researchers from the Silent Spring Institute say the grease-proof packaging often used by fast food chains contains potentially dangerous fluorinated chemicals, which can leak into the food.

In what they are calling the "most comprehensive analysis to date on the prevalence of highly fluorinated chemicals in fast food packaging in the United States," researchers say they tested 400 samples from 27 fast food chains for chemicals called PFASs (per- and polyfluoroalkyl substances), also called PFCs, which are often found in "nonstick, stain-resistant, and waterproof products, including carpeting, cookware, outdoor apparel, as well as food packaging."

Samples included paper wrappers, drink containers and paperboard.

"These chemicals have been linked with numerous health problems, so it's a concern that people are potentially exposed to them in food," said Laurel Schaider, an environmental chemist at Silent Spring Institute and the

Notes:

packaging／包装　harmful／有害な　suggest／示唆する　*Environmental Science & Technology Letters*／『エンバイロンメンタル・サイエンス・アンド・テクノロジー・レターズ』（環境科学技術に関する国際的討論雑誌）　the Silent Spring Institute／サイレントスプリング研究所（*Silent Spring*（『沈黙の春』）の著者Rachel Carsonに敬意を表して命名され，環境化学物質と女性の健康との関連性を特定し，公表している）　grease-proof／耐脂の（油をはじく）　potentially／潜在的に　fluorinated／フッ素化された　leak into ～／～に漏れ出る　comprehensive analysis／包括的な分析　to date／これまでで　prevalence／普及　test A for B／Bの有無を調べるためにAを検査する　PFASs (per- and polyfluoroalkyl substances)／ペルフルオロアルキルおよびポリフルオロアルキル物質　PFCs／ペルフルオロケミカルズ（生物の血液を汚染する有毒で残留性の高い過フッ素化合物類）　nonstick／こびりつかない　stain-resistant／しみがつきにくい　waterproof／防水性の　carpeting／敷物類　cookware／調理器具　outdoor apparel／アウトドア用衣類　A as well as B／BだけでなくAも　paper wrapper／包装紙　drink container／飲み物の容器　paperboard／板紙　be linked with ～／～と関連がある　It is a concern that ～／～は心配である　be exposed to ～／～に曝露する　environmental chemist／環境化学者

study's lead author. "Exposure to some PFASs has been associated with cancer, thyroid disease, immune suppression, low birth weight, and decreased fertility. Children are especially at risk for health effects because their developing bodies are more vulnerable to toxic chemicals.

Schaider added that about one out of every three children eat fast food every day.

In their analysis of fast food packaging, researchers said 20 percent of paperboard samples, including boxes for french fries and pizza, contained fluorine. Furthermore, Tex-Mex food packaging as well as bread and dessert wrapping was most likely to have fluorine.

In a more rigorous analysis of a subset of 20 samples, researchers found that "in general," samples were high in fluorine. They also contained PFASs.

Six of the samples contained a so-called long-chain PFAS called PFOA (perfluorooctanoic acid, also known as C8), which several U.S. manufacturers agreed to stop using after a 2011 review by the U.S. Food and Drug Administration.

Despite PFASs being phased out in the United States, they are still used in other countries. Some companies have been replacing them with shorter-chained PFAS compounds.

"The replacement compounds are equally persistent and have not been

Notes:

exposure／さらされること　be associated with ～／～と関連している　cancer／がん　thyroid disease／甲状腺疾患　immune suppression／免疫抑制　birth weight／出生時体重　fertility／生殖能力　be at risk for ～／～の危険がある　be vulnerable to ～／～の影響を受けやすい　toxic／毒性の　one out of every three children／3人に1人の子ども　fluorine／フッ素　furthermore／さらに　Tex-Mex food／テックス・メックス料理（テキサス風メキシコ料理）　be likely to ～／～である可能性が高い　rigorous／精密な, 厳密な　subset／全体の中の一部　"in general"／「たいていは」　long-chain PFAS／長鎖PFAS　PFOA (perfluorooctanoic acid)／ペルフルオロオクタン酸　manufacturer／製造業者, メーカー　review／見直し　the U.S. Food and Drug Administration／米国食品医薬品局　despite ～／～にも関わらず　phase ～ out／～を段階的に(使用)停止する　replace A with B／AをBに取り換える　shorter-chained PFAS compound／より短い原子連鎖のPFAS化合物　replacement compound／代替化合物　persistent／分解しにくい

shown to be safe for human health," says co-author Arlene Blum, founder of the Green Science Policy Institute. "That's why we need to reduce the use of the entire class of highly fluorinated compounds. The good news is there are non-fluorinated alternatives available."

Even if PFASs are phased out, researchers say they can still make their way into our bodies, either through the use of recycled materials or through accumulation in landfills, which could seep into groundwater.

"All PFASs, including the newer replacements, are highly resistant to degradation and will remain in the environment for a long time," says co-author Graham Peaslee, a physicist at the University of Notre Dame who developed the PIGE method to screen food wrappers. "Because of this, these highly fluorinated chemicals are not sustainable and should not be used in compostable products or any product that might end up in a landfill."

Notes:

co-author／共著者　the Green Science Policy Institute／グリーン科学政策研究所　That's why 〜／だから〜なのである　alternative／代替品　even if 〜／たとえ〜だとしても　make one's way into 〜／〜に入り込む　either A or B／AかBかいずれか　accumulation／蓄積　landfill／ごみ埋め立て地　seep into 〜／〜にしみ出る　groundwater／地下水　be resistant to 〜／〜に耐性のある，〜しにくい　degradation／分解　the University of Notre Dame／ノートルダム大学（米国インディアナ州にある名門私立大学）　the PIGE method／PIGE法（粒子線励起ガンマ線放出元素分析法という試料中の元素を同定する分析法で，PIGEはParticle Induced Gamma-ray Emissionの略語）　screen／検査する　because of 〜／〜のために，〜が原因で　sustainable／（環境破壊せず）持続的に利用可能な　compostable／堆肥にすることが可能な

練習問題

A 次の英文が本文の内容と一致する場合にはT，一致しない場合にはFを（　）内に記入しなさい。

1. (　) Due to extreme weather, water runoff has been increasing, but there is no evidence that this could lead to a large input of dangerous mercury into aquatic ecosystems.
2. (　) It is worrying that the amount of mercury in zooplankton could enormously increase, because that means we could also take in the toxic chemical through the food chain.
3. (　) In 2011, the U.S. FDA banned manufacturers from using highly fluorinated chemicals in food packaging.
4. (　) Fluorinated chemicals are highly toxic, but they are easily degradable and cause no environmental pollution.

B 音声を聴いて，次の英文の（　）内に適語を記入しなさい。　　track 19

1. Mosquitoes (　　) (　　) human and animal blood.
2. A lot of food (　　) (　　) in the garbage every day.
3. His family is (　　) (　　) (　　) heart disease.
4. The trade restrictions will be (　　) (　　) by 2020.

C 和文に合うように，（　）内の語句を並べかえて英文をつくりなさい。

1. 仕事と私生活のバランスを取るために，不要な残業を減らすべきだ。
   (unnecessary overwork, balance, to, work, on, should, back, private life, we, and, cut).

2. 青春時代をアメリカで過ごしたことは，彼のその後の人生に大きな影響を与えた。
   (had, his later life, his youth, the U.S., a, spending, impact, in, huge, on).

3. 肥満の人のほうが慢性的な疾患に罹りやすいことは確かである。
   (obese people, is, that, vulnerable, it, more, chronic diseases, certain, are, to).

4. 日本政府の報告書によると，2050年までには3人に1人が65歳以上になる。
   (every, by 2050, a report by the Japanese government, one, will, out of, over 65, three people, that, be, says).

D 次の英語に相当する日本語を下から選び，記号で答えなさい。
1. phytoplankton   ( )   2. zooplankton   ( )
3. photosynthesis   ( )   4. food chain   ( )
5. organic matter   ( )   6. stain-resistant   ( )
7. waterproof   ( )   8. thyroid disease   ( )
9. immune suppression   ( ) 10. fertility   ( )

a. 免疫抑制   b. 植物プランクトン   c. 動物プランクトン
d. しみがつきにくい e. 光合成   f. 甲状腺疾患
g. 食物連鎖   h. 生殖能力   i. 有機物
j. 防水性の

アジアの大都市が窒息!? 深刻化する大気汚染

Asian Cities Choking on Worsening Air Pollution

Voice of America, December 22, 2015

track 20

BANGKOK — Heavy smog on Tuesday shrouded the capitals of the world's two most populous countries. Air quality monitoring stations in Beijing and New Delhi displayed readings far exceeding the threshold for the highest-category hazardous level.

The Chinese capital on Monday and Tuesday was under its second-ever pollution red alert prompting Beijing's metropolitan government to order factories to reduce production or shut down, pull half the vehicles off the capital's roads and close schools.

The city's first red alert was issued on December 7.

In the early afternoon on Tuesday, air quality index machines in central Beijing showed readings in excess of 400 micrograms per cubic meter for PM2.5 (particles less than 2.5 micrometers in diameter, which can lodge in the lungs).

The issuing of red alerts, however, does not mean Beijing's air is actually

Notes:

choke on 〜／〜で息が詰まる，窒息する　worsen／悪化する　air pollution／大気汚染　Bangkok／バンコク（タイ王国の首都）　smog／スモッグ　shroud／覆う，包む　capital／首都　populous／人口の多い　monitor／監視する　Beijing／北京（中華人民共和国の首都）　New Delhi／ニューデリー（インドの首都）　display／表示する　reading／（計器などの）表示度数，示度　exceed／超える，上回る　threshold／境界，限界　hazardous／有害な　second-ever／これまでで2番目の　red alert／緊急非常事態，緊急警報　prompt A to 〜／Aに〜するよう促す　metropolitan government／（北京）市当局　reduce／低減する，減少させる　shut down／休業する　pull A off B／AをBから取り除く，締め出す　vehicle／車両　close／閉鎖する　issue／出す，発する　index／指標　in excess of 〜／〜を超過して　microgram／マイクログラム（100万分の1グラム）　per 〜／〜ごとに，〜につき　cubic meter／立法メートル　micrometer／マイクロメートル（100万分の1メートル）　diameter／直径　lodge／留まる　lung／肺

more polluted than it has been in the past.

"The reason that the municipal government decided to issue the red alert is to justify more radical measures to control the pollution level," said Yanzhong Huang, senior fellow for global health at the Council on Foreign Relations. "It turns out indeed that limiting the number of cars on the road actually brought down the level of pollution."

In India's capital, after a respite about a decade ago when anti-pollution measures led to improvements, the city is again choking on air considered the worst in the world, according to the World Health Organization (WHO).

"Studies have shown that in Delhi every third child has impaired lungs now. If you look at the number of premature deaths that get reported from different studies in this city that virtually works out to be one death per hour due to air pollution related diseases," said Anumita Roychowdhury, executive director for research and advocacy at the Center for Science and Environment in New Delhi.

The World Bank this year calculated that the shortened lifespans of people in India's cities due to air pollution is costing the country's economy $18 billion annually.

Notes:

in the past／従来，これまで　municipal government／市政(庁)，市役所　decide／決定する　justify／正当化する　radical／抜本的な，徹底的な　measures／対策，措置（通例は複数形）　senior fellow／上級研究員　the Council on Foreign Relations／外交問題評議会（米国に本拠を置く非営利の外交シンクタンク）　it turns out that 〜／〜であることがわかる　indeed／じつに，確かに　limit／制限する　the number of 〜／〜の数　bring down 〜／〜を下げる　respite／小休止，延期　decade／10年(間)　anti-pollution／汚染防止の　lead to 〜／〜をもたらす，〜につながる　improvement／改良，改善　consider 〜／〜とみなす，〜だと考える　according to 〜／〜によれば　the World Health Organization／世界保健機関（略称はWHO）　Delhi／デリー（インド北部の都市，かつてはインドの首都だった）　impaired／悪くなった，正常に機能しない　premature death／早死に　virtually／実質的には，事実上　work out to 〜／合わせて〜になる，〜に達する　due to 〜／〜が原因で，〜のために　related／関連のある，関係する　disease／疾病　executive director／事務局長，常任理事　advocacy／擁護　the Center for Science and Environment／科学環境センター（インドのニューデリーに本拠を置き，科学や環境問題などに関する情報の啓蒙を目的とする独立公益組織）　the World Bank／世界銀行　calculate／算出する　lifespan／寿命　cost／（費用が）かかる　billion／10億　annually／毎年，1年間に

"Right now during winter it's so visible. You can sense, you can smell that smog," Roychowdhury told VOA on Tuesday.

Little to show for vehicle bans, litigation

India's Supreme Court has banned through the end of March, registrations of large diesel luxury cars. The New Delhi government has ordered odd and even numbered vehicles to use roads on alternate days during the first half of January.

The Delhi High Court, which previously said that living in the Indian capital was akin to being in a "gas chamber," on Monday declared an emergency. Two judges of the court directed all concerned authorities to follow existing rules, chastised traffic police for being ineffective in reducing road congestion and ordered officials to ensure particulate matter levels not exceed 60 micrograms per cubic meter per day for the particularly lethal PM2.5 and 100 micrograms per cubic meter per day for PM10.

The WHO considers any level above 25 micrograms as unsafe.

The U.S. Embassy in New Delhi late Tuesday morning recorded the air quality index at a hazardous 534.

The judicial intervention in India comes after public interest litigation initiated as far back as 20 years ago.

"The reason why the courts get involved is when the civil society is angry

---

Notes:

right now／ちょうど今　visible／見てわかる,（見た目に）明らかな　sense／感じる, 気づく　smell／においがする, においがわかる　ban／禁止　litigation／訴訟　Supreme Court／最高裁判所　registration／登録　odd and even numbered vehicles／（ナンバープレートが）奇数と偶数の車両　alternate／交互に起こる, 交替の　previously／以前には　be akin to ～／～と似ている　"gas chamber"／「ガス(処刑)室」　declare／宣言する, 言明する　emergency／緊急事態, 非常事態　judge／裁判官, 判事　concerned authorities／（関係）当局, 所轄官庁　chastise／強く非難する　ineffective／効果のない, 無駄な　congestion／（交通）渋滞　ensure／確実にする　particulate matter／粒子状物質　lethal／死をもたらす　unsafe／安全でない　U.S. Embassy／米国大使館　judicial／司法上の, 裁判上の　intervention／仲裁, 調停　come after ～／～の後に来る　public interest litigation／公益訴訟　initiate／始める, 起こす　as far back as ～／～まで遡って　the reason why ～／～の理由　get involved／関わる, 関係する　civil／民間(人)の, 一般人の　be angry about ～／～に立腹している, 怒っている

about an issue and they use the public interest litigation instrument to go to the court to seek relief," explained Roychowdhury. "In response to that public interest litigation the courts respond. So it is not that the judges just suddenly intervene on their own."

The central government's transport minister, Nitin Gadkari, has vowed to cut Delhi's pollution by building a ring road so trucks will not have to drive through the capital. He also wants more vehicles to use ethanol fuel. But the minister acknowledges this will not solve the bad air problem in Delhi because burning farm waste and construction dust also contribute.

Problems in Dhaka, Tehran

In Dhaka, the world's fastest growing mega-city where at least 15 million people are residing, traffic congestion and smoke from brick kilns create pollution blamed for killing thousands of residents every year and causing between 80 million and 230 million cases annually of respiratory diseases, according to the Bangladesh Ministry of Environment and Forests.

"During the winter it's dry and there's a lot of construction," thus the air pollution is worse, said associate professor of chemistry Mominul Islam who answered the phone Tuesday at the University of Dhaka's air quality research and monitoring center.

The center, as well as the Bangladesh Ministry of Environment, however, have no equipment to record PM2.5 readings, according to the professor, thus there is no way to gauge whether Dhaka's air is currently worse than Beijing's or Delhi's.

"We hope to have equipment online from February," he said.

A high pollution alert also prompted Iranian authorities in Tehran, Isfahan and Arak, to close all schools for two days from Sunday. It was the first such order since 2010.

The PM2.5 levels recorded Sunday and Monday in Tehran were in the unhealthy range, but far superior to those of Beijing and New Delhi.

Canned air for sale

Across the region authorities are still grappling with how to combat the pollution in the long run.

"Even in the case of China where we've seen the top leaders themselves increasingly committed to pollution control there's no consensus on how to effectively address the problem," Huang, a professor at Seton Hall University who just returned from Beijing, told VOA. "And, of course, in Delhi, India you face similar challenges on how to handle the dilemma between economic development and environmental pollution."

Well-heeled Chinese are purchasing high-quality imported air purifiers for their homes and offices. But those units are too expensive for many Chinese who have resorted to rigging up makeshift units by attaching glass-fiber

---

Notes:

there is no way to ～／～する方法がない，～できない　gauge／判断する，評価する　whether ～／～かどうか　currently／現在，今のところ　online／（装置が通信回線などに接続されて）作動中で　Iranian／イランの　such／そのような　superior to ～／～よりすぐれている　canned／缶詰にした　for sale／売り物の，売りに出した　grapple with ～／～に取り組む　how to ～／～する方法　combat／戦う　in the long run／長い目で見れば，結局は　in the case of ～／～の場合，～については　commit／約束する，言質を与える　consensus／コンセンサス，統一見解　address／取り組む　Seton Hall University／シートンホール大学（米国ニュージャージー州に所在するカトリック系の名門私立大学）　of course／もちろん，確かに　face／直面する　challenge／課題，難問　handle／扱う，処理する　dilemma／ジレンマ，板挟み　well-heeled／金持ちの　purchase／購入する　air purifier／空気清浄機　unit／装置，設備　too ～ for A／Aにとってあまりに～　resort to ～／（最後の手段として）～に訴える，頼る　rig up／急ごしらえする，ありあわせで作る　makeshift／一時しのぎの，間に合わせの　glass-fiber／グラスファイバー，ガラス繊維

⁹⁵ filters to household fans.

A Canadian company, Vitality Air, which began bottling Rocky Mountain air as a joke, now claims to have sold thousands of cans in China for up to $28 each.

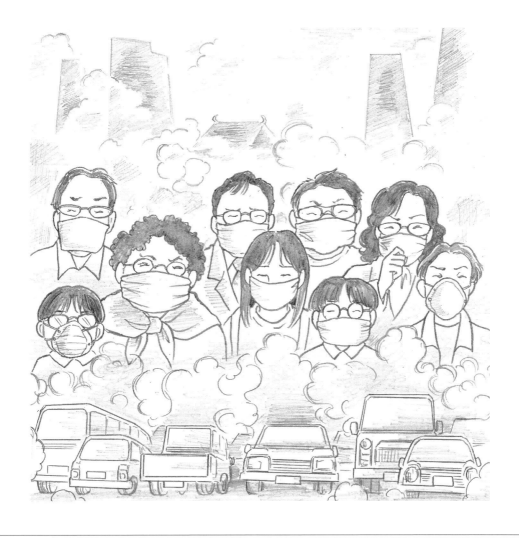

Notes:

household／家庭用の，ありふれた　Vitality Air／バイタリティー・エアー（カナダのアルバータ州エドモントンに本拠を置く，新鮮な空気を販売する会社）　bottle／びん詰めにする　Rocky Mountain／ロッキー山脈（北米西部の大山系）　joke／冗談，しゃれ　claim／主張する，断言する　up to 〜／〜まで

練習問題

A 次の英文が本文の内容と一致する場合にはT，一致しない場合にはFを（　）内に記入しなさい。

1. (　) According to a senior fellow at the Council on Foreign Relations, limiting the number of cars on the road reduced the level of air pollution.
2. (　) The Delhi High Court said that living in New Delhi was similar to being in a gas chamber.
3. (　) In Dhaka, Teheran, burning farm waste and construction dust create air pollution.
4. (　) Rich Chinese people are now purchasing high-quality imported air purifiers for their homes and offices.

B 音声を聴いて，次の英文の（　）内に適語を記入しなさい。　　track 21

1. Savings of ¥500 a day will (　　) (　　) (　　) more than ¥180,000 in a year.
2. I (　　) very (　　) (　　) what you did to me.
3. There (　　) (　　) way (　　) solve the problem.
4. We offer you (　　) (　　) 40％ discount of all of our products.

C 和文に合うように，（　）内の語句を並べかえて英文をつくりなさい。

1. 交通渋滞のせいで，私は会議に遅れて到着した。
   (to, due, the meeting, late, I, heavy, arrived, traffic, to).

2. ネットワークのファイヤーウォールは，ビルの警備システムに似ている。
   (akin, a network firewall, security system, is, the building, to).

3. 顧客の苦情に応えて，私たちは詫状を送った。
   (a, in, sent, customer's, response, an apology letter, to, complaint, we).

4. 当局は幼児虐待の問題に取り組んできた。
   (abuse, grappled, the authorities, the issues, with, have, child, of).

D 次の英語に相当する日本語を下から選び，記号で答えなさい。

1. bronchus　　　　（　）　2. inhalation　　　　（　）
3. exhalation　　　（　）　4. respiration　　　　（　）
5. wheeze　　　　　（　）　6. pneumonia　　　　（　）
7. dyspnea　　　　（　）　8. asthma　　　　　　（　）
9. cough　　　　　（　）　10. trachea　　　　　（　）

a. 呼吸困難　　　　b. 喘息　　　　　　c. 喘鳴(ぜんめい)
d. 呼気　　　　　　e. 呼吸　　　　　　f. 吸入
g. 気管　　　　　　h. 肺炎　　　　　　i. 気管支
j. 咳

Unit 10 認知症のリスクを下げるのは？

> **Strong Heart, Better Education Shown to Lower Dementia Risk**
>
> Voice of America, December 28, 2016

🔊 track 22

As the elderly population continues to grow globally, the number of people who will suffer (1) dementia also will increase. The question is, by how much?

The World Health Organization estimates that close to 50 million people have been diagnosed (2) dementia, with more than half living in low- and middle-income countries.

Although dementia mainly affects older people, it is not a normal part of aging. (3)As researchers find out more about the causes of dementia, they are also finding ways they can help reduce its prevalence.

Watch: Good Heart Health, Education Equals Lower Risk For Dementia

For example, numerous studies show that what's good for the heart is also good for the brain. (4)Physical activity and a healthy diet keep the heart pumping and blood flowing to the brain. Good blood flow keeps the brain functioning, and has been shown to reduce the risk of dementia.

Brains shrink with age, but (5)studies cited by the Alzheimer's Society of the U.K. showed that aerobic exercise not only increases the heart rate, but also enlarges the hippocampus, the key area of the brain involved in memory. In one study, a year of aerobic exercise by older adults proved (6) be the equivalent of reversing one to two years of age-related shrinkage.

(7)Researchers also have found a link between higher education and a reduction in dementia. Studies continue to look at the way exercise, diet, social and mental stimulation, and other factors influence the development of dementia, Alzheimer's being the most common form of this disease.

Dr. Kenneth Langa at the University of Michigan focuses his research on dementia. He was the co-investigator of a study of 20,000 adults in the United States over a 12-year period, and was the lead investigator of a supplemental study on the risk factors and prevalence of dementia in this group.

"We found that the prevalence of dementia declined significantly between 2000 and 2012, from about 11.5 percent down to about 9 percent," Langa said.

Langa attributes the decline in dementia to better treatments for high blood pressure, diabetes and obesity — treatments that keep the cardiovascular system healthy and lower incidents of stroke. He also says increases in education levels play a role.

In the U.S., education levels rose over the past two decades, according to data gathered by Langa. A larger percentage of people graduated from high school, and more people received college educations. Langa's study showed that (8)even a slight increase in the level of education seems to have an impact in reducing the risk of dementia.

"This suggests that a 75-year-old today has a lower risk of having dementia today than a 75-year-old 10 or 20 years ago," he said.

But the numbers were still significant because (9   ) the large number of older adults.

"What we found was that for adults in the United States, ages 65 and older, about 3 to 5 percent of them who were 65 to 74 had dementia, and that went up to almost 30 percent for those who are 85 and older," Langa said. "So almost one in three had dementia in our study."

Even without a breakthrough in treatment, Langa says (10)[things, the risk, that, decrease, are, appears, can, there, it]. However, he says, more work needs to be done to keep dementia trends declining.

The supplemental study was published in *the Journal of the American Medical Association*.

Notes:

dementia／認知症　the number of ～／～の数　the World Health Organization／世界保健機関（略称はWHO）　estimate／推定する　close to ～／（数値が）～に近い，およそ～　low- and middle-income／低・中所得の　affect／影響を与える　aging／高齢化，老化　find out ～／～を見つけ出す，突き止める　reduce／減少させる　prevalence／罹患率　equal／生み出す，招く　for example／例えば　numerous／非常に多くの　keep A ～ing／Aを～させておく　pump／鼓動する　blood／血液　shrink／萎縮する　cite／引用する　the Alzheimer's Society of the U. K.／英国アルツハイマー病協会　aerobic exercise／有酸素運動　not only A but also B／AだけでなくBもまた　heart rate／心拍数　enlarge／拡大する　hippocampus／（脳の）海馬　involved in ～／～に関わりのある　equivalent／同等物　reverse／逆にする　shrinkage／萎縮　between A and B／AとBの間　reduction／減少　look at ～／～を検討する　stimulation／刺激　influence／影響を及ぼす　supplemental／補足の，追加の　decline／減少する　significantly／かなり，著しく　attribute A to B／AをBに帰する，AをBのせいにする　treatment／治療　high blood pressure／高血圧（hypertension）　diabetes／糖尿病　obesity／（病的な）肥満　cardiovascular system／心（臓）血管系，循環（器）系　incident／出来事　stroke／発作，(脳)卒中　play a role／役割を果たす　according to ～／～によれば　gather／収集する　slight／わずかな　seem to ～／～するように思われる　significant／かなり大きな　up to ～／（数値が）～まで　those who ～／～な人たち　breakthrough／飛躍的進歩　trend／傾向，方向　*the Journal of the American Medical Association*（JAMA）／『ジャーナル・オブ・ジ・アメリカン・メディカル・アソシエーション』（米国医師会が発行する学術雑誌）

練習問題

A 本文中の (1)(2)(6)(9) に適語を入れなさい（音声を参考にしてもよい）。
(1) (　　　　)　(2) (　　　　)　(6) (　　　　)　(9) (　　　　)

B (10) が「そのリスクを減らすかもしれないものがあるようだ」という意味になるように [　　　] 内の語句を並べかえなさい（音声を参考にしてもよい）。

C 下線部 (3) (4) (5) (7) (8) を日本語に直しなさい。

(3)

(4)

(5)

(7)

(8)

D 次の説明に合う語を英文中から選びなさい。

(11) an illness that affects the brain and memory, and makes you gradually lose the ability to think and behave normally (   )

(12) the part of the body inside the head that controls thoughts, feelings, and movements (   )

(13) the action or process of teaching someone especially in a school, college, or university (   )

(14) a disease in which the body cannot control the amount of sugar in the blood (   )

(15) the condition of being too fat in a way that is dangerous to your health (   )

Review (Unit 6〜Unit 9)

A 英文の（　）内に入る語を下から選んで記入し，英文を日本語に直しなさい。

1. You used (　　) live in Seattle, didn't you? (Unit 6)

2. A new car is out (　　) the question. It's too expensive. (Unit 7)

3. This table can serve (　　) a desk. (Unit 8)

4. You may want to quit school now, but (　　) the long run, you'll regret it. (Unit 9)

> as,　in,　of,　to

B 和文に合うように，（　）内の語句を並べかえて英文をつくりなさい。

1. 何千人もの人々がそのウイルスに感染してしまった。(Unit 6)
   (the virus, people, with, been, of, infected, thousands, have).

2. 消防車が到着するときまでには，家全体が炎に包まれていた。(Unit 7)
   (was, arrived, the whole house, fire, the time, the fire engines, by, on).

3. 身長が低いという事実にもかかわらず，彼は素晴らしいバレーボール選手だ。(Unit 8)
   (short, he, an excellent volleyball player, is, that, he, despite, is, the fact).

4. 彼らが10年間浮気をしてきたということがわかった。(Unit 9)
   (an affair, been, for ten years, out, having, turned, they'd, that, it).

C 次の英語に相当する日本語を下から選び，記号で答えなさい。

1. ignorance　　　　（　）　2. prevention　　　　（　）
3. treatment　　　　（　）　4. suicide　　　　　（　）
5. photosynthesis　（　）　6. emission　　　　（　）
7. disposal　　　　（　）　8. lung　　　　　　（　）
9. immune　　　　 （　）　10. litigation　　　　（　）

> a. 免疫　　　　b. 治療　　　　c. 訴訟
> d. 処分　　　　e. 無知　　　　f. 予防
> g. 肺　　　　　h. 自殺　　　　i. 光合成
> j. 排出

Unit 11 性犯罪のない大学をめざせ!

US Universities Work to Prevent Sexual Abuse

Voice of America, October 02, 2015

track 23

WASHINGTON — As college students headed back to campus across the U.S. this fall, many encountered something new: mandatory workshops designed to prevent sexual abuse.

Faced with an increase of reported sexual assaults on college campuses, many U.S. universities launched programs aimed at promoting student awareness of sexual violence.

In Washington DC, George Washington University, American University and Georgetown University are just a few of the institutions implementing programs to provide students with tools to help prevent sexual assault and resources for victims.

The latest survey from the Association of American Universities found that 20 percent of students reported sexual assault last year alone. That has prompted universities to take steps to prevent such cases.

Notes:

prevent／防止する　sexual abuse／性的虐待　head back to 〜／〜に戻る　encounter／思いがけなく出会う、はじめて見る　mandatory／強制力のある　workshop／研修会　designed to 〜／〜することを目的とした　faced with 〜／〜と直面して　reported／報告された　sexual assault／性的暴行　launch／始める　aimed at 〜／〜を目的とした　promote／高める　awareness／意識　sexual violence／性的暴力　Washington DC／ワシントンD. C.（米国の首都）　George Washington University (GWU)／ジョージ・ワシントン大学（ワシントンD. C.にある私立大学）　American University／アメリカン大学 (AU)（ワシントンD. C. にある私立大学）　Georgetown University／ジョージタウン大学（ワシントンD. C. 近郊のジョージタウンにある私立大学）　institution／（教育的)機関　implement／実施する　provide A with B／AにBを提供する　tool／手段　resources／援助　victim／被害者　latest／最新の　survey／調査　the Association of American Universities／米国大学協会　report／報告する　〜 alone／〜だけで　prompt A to 〜／Aに〜するよう促す　take steps／対策を講ずる

Robert D. Hradsky, Assistant Vice President of Campus Life at American University, says effective programs to prevent sexual violence must begin the moment students first arrive on campus for orientation.

"In the very first week, when students arrive on campus, they go through a 90-minute training called 'Empower A.U.' that also goes over issues around interpersonal sexual violence, consent, and myths around relationship violence," said Hradsky.

"We try to give students the tools they need in particular to intervene when they see that someone might be in harm's way", he said.

Increase in sexual assaults

Over the last three years the number of reported incidents of sexual assault at American University increased, from 36 cases in 2012-13 to 61 in 2014-15.

In response, the school crafted clear standards for incidents of sexual assaults, and procedures for providing help to victims.

"The most immediate concern is ensuring the safety of the survivor," Hradsky told VOA. "We want to make sure that the survivor understands all the resources, so that if they need medical care they know where they can receive it. If they are interested in collecting evidence in the event that they may want to pursue criminal charges, they understand how to do that

Notes:

case／事例 Assistant Vice President of Campus Life／学生生活支援部部長補佐 effective／効果的な the moment ～／～するとすぐに go through ～／～を終える called ～／～とよばれている empower／能力を与える 'Empower A.U.'／『エンパワー・アメリカン大学』（アメリカン大学（A.U.）の新入生に性的暴力防止について指導するためのプログラム） go over ～／～を検討する issue／重要な点, 問題点 interpersonal／個人間で起こる consent／同意 myth／根拠のない社会通念 relationship violence／カップル間の暴力, 恋愛関係相手の暴力 in particular／とくに intervene／介入する in harm's way／危険な状態に the number of ～／～の数 incident／事件 in response／（前文を受けて）それに応じて craft／念入りに作る standard／基準 procedure／手順, 手続き immediate concern／当面の関心事 ensure／確保する survivor／助かった人 make sure that ～／確実に～する so that ～／その結果～, だから～ medical care／治療 be interested in ～／～に関心がある collect／集める evidence／証拠, 証言 in the event that ～／万一～の場合には pursue／求める criminal charges／刑事責任 how to ～／～する方法

and where to go, and we help them get there," he said.

35　Additionally, the university created a Sexual Assault Working Group, charged with reviewing university efforts on issues of interpersonal and sexual violence including sexual assault, dating, and domestic violence and stalking.

Hradsky says the group of 13 students takes part in decisions on how 40　sexual assault cases are managed. "We are working very closely with all of students' representatives to help to inform our approach and be a part of the solution," he said.

Bringing abuse out in the open

Across town, George Washington University this fall mandated sexual 45　assault prevention training for incoming freshmen and graduate students, followed by an online program later in the summer.

"Our strategy has been and will continue to be having a comprehensive, multifaceted approach to sexual assault awareness education," said Dr. Konwerski, GWU Dean of Student Affairs in a press release published on 50　the university's website. "This summer we will continue this approach with some new offerings."

The program was first proposed by GW Students Against Sexual Assault (SASA), an association specifically formed to combat sexual assault.

Notes:

additionally／さらに　Sexual Assault Working Group／性的暴力特別調査委員会　charged with ～ing／～することを任されている　review／調査する　efforts on ～／～に対する取り組み，努力　including ～／～を含む　dating violence／デート・バイオレンス（デート中の性暴力）　domestic violence／ドメスティック・バイオレンス（配偶者や恋人など親密な関係にある，またはあった者からの暴力）　stalking／つきまとい，ストーカー行為　take part in ～／～に参加する　manage／対処する　closely／密接に　representative／代表者　inform／知らせる　approach／取り組み方　solution／解決　bring ～ out in the open／～を公表する　mandate／命じる　prevention training／防止訓練　incoming／入ってくる　freshman／新入生　graduate student／大学院生　followed by ～／～，続いて～がある　strategy／方略　comprehensive／包括的な　multifaceted／多角的な　Dean of Student Affairs／学生部長　press release／報道発表　publish／公表する　offering／講義科目　propose／提案する　Students Against Sexual Assault (SASA)／性的暴行に反対する学生の会　association／団体　specifically／特別に　formed／結成された　combat／闘う

Lauren Courtney studies political science and pre-law at GWU, and serves as director of Policy and Community Outreach at SASA. Courtney says the program features conversations about drinking alcohol, campus safety, living in a city, as well as sexual violence.

"The university really wanted to talk about mental health, making sure that students are safe and not drinking too much, but the university didn't want to talk about sexual assault," Courtney told VOA. "For a long time it just has been a norm for the university to pretend that sexual assault doesn't happen on campus because it's a huge liability. A university's worst nightmare is to have a scandal," she said.

Data from the AAU study shows that more than 1 in 5 female undergrads at top schools reported suffering a sexual attack, but Courtney believes the real number is bigger. "I think that sexual assault always has been this big. People knew that it was going on and their studies showed that it was going on, but people were so discouraged from reporting," Courtney added.

All university students who have experienced sexual assault have the right to report the abuse if they so choose. Once a report is made, a U.S. law called Title IX mandates that the school provide treatment.

"They have to find ways to help the survivors still function at the university," said Lauren Courtney. "That could mean having a legal process at the university to try the students of sexual assault and after it convicted they could be suspended, and/or forced to leave the university."

Notes:

political science／政治学　pre-law／法科大学院入学準備コース　serve as ～／～の役割を果たす　director／理事　Policy and Community Outreach／方針と地域社会への奉仕活動に関する分科委員会　feature／特色にする　A as well as B／BだけでなくAも　mental health／心の健康　norm／規範　pretend／ふりをする　huge／非常に大きな　liability／不都合なこと　nightmare／悪夢のような出来事　scandal／不祥事, スキャンダル　more than ～／～より多い　female／女性の　undergrad／大学生, 学部学生　suffer／経験する, 被る　sexual attack／性的暴行　go on／続く　discourage A from ～ing／Aが～することを思いとどまらせる　add／付け加える　right／権利　so／そのように　choose／望む, 決める　once ～／いったん～すると　a U.S. law called Title IX／教育改正法第9編と呼ばれている米国の法律（連邦が財政支援する学校などの教育活動における性差別の禁止を規定）　treatment／措置　still／今でも　function／本来の活動をする　legal process／訴訟手続き　try／裁判にかける　after it (is) convicted／それが有罪判決を下された後　suspend／停学させる　(be) forced to ～／強制的に～される

Robert Hradsky pointed out that sexual violence is now on the public agenda, and that people are speaking more publicly because of the national visibility. Hradsky said years ago when he was in school, people didn't speak about sexual assault.

"That is absolutely a difference," Hradsky said. "So, back then, you generally didn't talk about it a whole lot. Now with all this national visibility, clearly it's a part of the everyday conversation in campus."

At American University, speaking about the problem of sexual assault is becoming more common – an important step to preventing it, says Hradsky. "It is better to show the problem than to pretend we do not see it, because it exists."

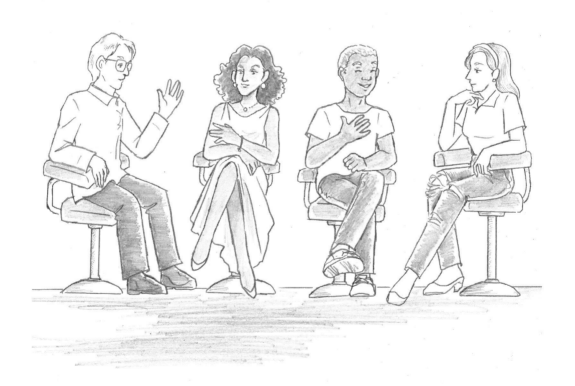

Notes:
point out that 〜／〜ということを指摘する　public agenda／周知の議題　publicly／公然と　because of 〜／〜の理由で　national／全国的な　visibility／注目度　absolutely／絶対的な　back then／その当時は　not 〜 a whole lot／あまり〜でない　common／普通の　exist／存在する

練習問題

A 次の英文が本文の内容と一致する場合にはT，一致しない場合にはFを（ ）内に記入しなさい。

1. (　) The number of reported sexual assault incidents at American University is decreasing every year thanks to the sexual abuse prevention workshops.
2. (　) George Washington University set up a student association which convicts and punishes students of sexual assault.
3. (　) To admit that sexual assaults are happening on campus has been the shame to universities.
4. (　) Bringing the sexual assault problem out in the open is a significant step towards its prevention.

B 音声を聴いて，次の英文の（　）内に適語を記入しなさい。　　track 24

1. He (　) (　) (　) his job.
2. My brother (　) (　) six-week-long training for a full marathon.
3. Many students (　) (　) (　) the weekend workshop.
4. The leader (　) (　) (　) make a difficult decision.

C 和文に合うように，（　）内の語句を並べかえて英文をつくりなさい。

1. 高熱の後に発疹が出た。
   (by, fever, was, the, the rash, high, followed).

2. 政府は環境汚染を防止するための緊急の措置を講じた。
   (steps, pollution, the government, urgent, to, environmental, took, prevent).

3. 彼らは彼女が正当な理由なく学校をやめるのを思いとどまらせようとした。
   (discourage, tried, with, her, leaving school, they, no reasonable excuse, from, to).

4. 学生に学術的な文章を書く技術を身につけさせる授業を君は受けるべきだ。
   (provides, take, academic writing skills, with, the course, you, which, should, students).

D 次の英語に相当する日本語を下から選び，記号で答えなさい。

1. spousal abuse （　） 2. intimidation （　）
3. network abuse （　） 4. fraud （　）
5. larceny （　） 6. indecent exposure （　）
7. stalking （　） 8. malicious mischief （　）
9. sexual harassment （　） 10. plagiarism （　）

a. ネットワーク不正使用　　b. 公然わいせつ　　c. 剽窃
d. 故意による器物損壊　　　e. 脅迫　　　　　　f. 詐欺
g. セクハラ　　　　　　　　h. 配偶者虐待　　　i. 窃盗
j. ストーカー行為

Unit 12 生かされない教訓　日本の過労死問題

Japan Overwork Deaths Among Young Show Lessons Unlearned

Voice of America, October 21, 2016
Associated Press

🔊 track 25

TOKYO — Matsuri Takahashi's dream career at Japan's top ad agency, Dentsu, ended with her suicide as her overtime pushed past 100 hours a month.

"I'm emotionless and only wish to sleep," she wrote, exhausted and
5　depressed, in a Twitter post in October 2015, six months after starting the job. On Christmas day, the 24-year-old leaped from a dormitory balcony, leaving behind a last email to her mother saying her work and life had become unbearable.

Takahashi's was not the first "karoshi," or death from overwork at Dentsu,
10　a company notorious for demanding long hours from its employees.

Despite efforts over the past two decades to cut back on overwork, karoshi* still causes hundreds of deaths and illnesses every year in Japan, affecting all sorts of workers, from elite "salarymen and career women" employees like Takahashi to IT technicians and manual laborers.

（＊：ここでは書き手はkaroshi＝overworkのニュアンスでとらえていると考えられる）

Notes:

overwork death／過労死　unlearned／生かされていない　Associated Press／AP通信社（世界的な通信網を持つ米国の大手通信社）　ad agency／広告代理店　Dentsu／電通　end with ～／～で終わる　suicide／自殺　overtime／残業　push past ～／～を大幅に越える　emotionless／感情のない，無感動な　exhausted／疲れ果てた　depressed／うつ状態の　Twitter post／ツイッターの投稿　leap from ～／～から飛び降りる　leave behind ～／～を残す　unbearable／耐え難い　be notorious for ～／～（悪いこと）で有名な　long hours／長時間（労働）　despite ～／～にも関わらず　decade／10年間　cut back on ～／～を減らす　hundreds of ～／何百もの～　IT technician／IT技術者　manual laborer／肉体労働者

15　In August 2015, labor authorities caught Dentsu exceeding its own 70-hour monthly maximum overtime limit and ordered it to cut back.

Asked for comment, Dentsu said that as of October 2015, nobody was reporting overtime exceeding 70 hours. It now limits overtime to 50 hours a month. "We will keep trying to manage work appropriately, to curb long
20　hours of work and maintain employees' health," Dentsu told The Associated Press in a statement.

But at Dentsu and many other companies, much overtime goes unreported, labor officials say.

On top of the 40-hour work week the Labor Standards Law sets for most
25　workers, as an exception that serves as a loophole companies can establish voluntary ceilings for overtime. That makes the law toothless, experts say.

In Japan's male-dominated, hierarchical corporate world, company interests tend to come first. Employees, especially young, foreign or female workers, are ill-placed to resist pressure from higher-ups to work extra-long
30　hours or take on too much work. Older workers who retire from permanent positions with full benefits often are replaced by part-timers or chronically overworked contractors who likewise have little leverage and no union representation.

"Overtime is supposed to be for unanticipated occasions, but in Japan, it's
35　become expected as part of daily duties that nobody can refuse," said

Notes:
labor authorities／労働関係の当局, ここでは労働局のこと　catch A ～ing／Aが～しているのを見つける　exceed／越える　as of ～／～現在　limit A to B／AをBに制限する　keep ～ing／～し続ける　appropriately／適切に　curb／抑制する, 歯止めをかける　statement／声明　go unreported／報告されないままになる　on top of ～／～に加えて　the Labor Standard Law／労働基準法　serve as ～／～の役割を果たす　loophole／抜け穴, 逃げ道　voluntary ceiling for ～／～に対する任意の上限　toothless／実効性を欠く, 骨抜きの　male-dominated／男性優位の　hierarchical／階層的な　corporate world／企業社会　tend to ～／～しがちである　come first／最優先である　ill-placed／弱い立場に置かれた　higher-up／上司　extra-long hours／極端に長い時間　take on ～／～を引き受ける　permanent position／常勤職　with full benefits／手当の満額受給で　part-timer／非常勤で働く人, パートタイマー　chronically／慢性的に　contractor／契約社員　likewise／同じく, 同様に　leverage／（目的達成のための）影響力, 力　union representation／組合代表　be supposed to ～／～することになっている　unanticipated／予期されない　occasion／場合, 時　daily duty／日常の職務

Kansai University professor Koji Morioka, an expert on labor issues. "People are chronically working long hours because they have too much work to do as staff sizes have shrunk."

Prime Minister Shinzo Abe's government wants companies to drastically cut working hours to enable men to help out more at home and create more job opportunities for women. But that strategy, dubbed "womenomics," appears to be making little headway.

Takahashi's case became public after the government recently recognized her suicide as "karoshi."

"I'm on duty again Saturday-Sunday. I just want to die," she tweeted in November 2015. By December she was getting only two hours of sleep a day.

Asked during parliamentary questioning about Takahashi's death, the third officially acknowledged case of "karoshi" at Dentsu, Minister of Health, Labor and Welfare Yasuhisa Shiozaki threatened harsh action against the company, which dominates advertising for both companies and the government.

"It is extremely regrettable that the lesson was not learned and yet another young employee ended up committing suicide at the same company because of long working hours," he said.

There is growing recognition that efforts to curb overwork are failing and that the pressure increasingly is affecting younger workers, said Emiko Teranishi, who founded a group for karoshi victims' families after her husband, a chef, died of overwork.

Notes:
staff size／人員　shrink／縮小する　drastically／抜本的に　enable A to ～／Aが～できるようにする　job opportunity／雇用機会　strategy／戦略　dub／呼ぶ　"womenomics"／「ウーマノミクス」　appear to ～／～するように見える　make headway／前進する, 進展する　become public／公になる　on duty／勤務中で　parliamentary questioning／国会での質疑　Minister of Health, Labor and Welfare／厚生労働大臣　threaten harsh action against ～／～に対して厳しい措置を取ることを示唆する　both A and B／AもBも両方とも　regrettable／遺憾な, 悔やまれる　end up ～ing／結局～する　because of ～／～が原因で　found／設立する　die of ～／～が原因で死ぬ

A survey of 10,000 companies published in Japan's first white paper on karoshi, released this month, found that overtime at more than 20 percent exceeded the 80-hour-per-month threshold for overwork.

In 2015 alone, 93 suicides and attempted suicides were officially recognized as overwork deaths and eligible for compensation and 96 deaths from heart attacks, strokes and other illnesses were linked to overwork, it said. It listed 1,515 cases of workers or families seeking compensation for overwork-related mental problems.

More than half of Japanese workers give up taking paid vacations, while more than one in five Japanese work an average of 49 hours or longer each week, compared to 16.4 percent in the U.S., 12.5 percent in Britain and 10.1 percent in Germany.

Many Japanese karoshi victims were men in their 30s and 40s in managerial positions entailing no legal limits on overtime.

That includes a 40-year-old nuclear engineer at Kansai Electric Power in Tsuruga, western Japan, who hanged himself in April. Regulators found he had logged up to 200 hours of overtime a month.

Highlighting another lapse in oversight, workers in Japan's vocational training programs for foreign workers are among the most vulnerable.

A 27-year-old Philippine man, Joey Tocnang, died of heart failure in April

Notes:

survey／調査　publish／掲載する　white paper／白書（政府の公式報告書）　release／発表する　more than ～／～より多い　threshold for ～／～の限度, 許容範囲　～alone／～だけで　attempted suicide／自殺未遂　be eligible for ～／～を受ける資格がある　compensation／賠償金　heart attack／心臓発作　stroke／（脳）卒中　be linked to ～／～と関連している　mental problems／精神的疾患　give up ～ing／～することを諦める　paid vacation／有給休暇　compared to ～／～と比較すると, に対して　managerial position／管理職　entail／（必然的結果として）～を伴う　nuclear engineer／原子力技師　Kansai Electric Power／関西電力　Tsuruga／敦賀（美浜発電所のある福井県敦賀半島のこと）　hang oneself／首を吊る　regulator／監査機関　log／記録に残す　up to ～／～まで　highlight／大きく取り上げる, 強調する　lapse in oversight／監督が行き届いていないこと　vocational training program／職業訓練プログラム　vulnerable／弱い立場の　heart failure／心不全

2014 while participating in a government-sponsored training program at a die-casting factory in central Japan's Gifu prefecture. His monthly overtime exceeding 120 hours was recognized as the cause of his death just months before he was due to finish the three-year program.

Growing official recognition seems not to have altered the tendency for long hours to trump work-life balance.

Dentsu's taxing regime has persisted since the lean years just after World War II, when then-company president Hideo Yoshida, dubbed the "demon of advertising" devised his "10 rules of work."

At the top of the list: "Create work for yourself; don't wait for work to be assigned to you." Another says, "Never give up, even if you might be killed."

A landmark Supreme Court decision in 2003 recognized the 1991 suicide of a 24-year-old Dentsu radio advertising worker as karoshi. A 30-year-old Dentsu employee who died of illness three years ago also was recognized as an overwork victim.

"Someone tell me why my daughter had to die," Takahashi's mother Yukimi said after winning an undisclosed amount of compensation for her daughter, whose name means "Festival."

"I wish someone had taken steps sooner when she was still alive."

Notes:

participate in ～／～に参加する　die-casting／ダイカスト（溶かした金属に圧力をかけて金属製の鋳型に注入する鋳造法）　be due to ～／～することになっている　seem to ～／～であるように見える，思われる　alter／変える　tendency for A to ～／Aが～する傾向　trump／～を凌ぐ　taxing regime／社員を酷使する企業体制　persist／根強く残る　lean years／貧しい時代　then-company president／当時の会社社長　demon／鬼　devise／考え出す　"10 rules of work"／「鬼十則」（電通社員の行動規範）　be assigned to ～／～に割り当てられる　even if ～／たとえ～だとしても　landmark／画期的な　Supreme Court decision／最高裁判所の判決　undisclosed／公表されていない　amount of compensation／賠償額　I wish S 過去完了形／Sが～だったらよかったのに　take steps／対策を講じる

練習問題

A 次の英文が本文の内容と一致する場合にはT，一致しない場合にはFを（　）内に記入しなさい。

1. (　) Deaths and illnesses caused by overwork are found only in workers of particular job types.
2. (　) In Japan's corporate world, it is primarily female workers who find it difficult to resist pressure from their bosses to work extra-long hours.
3. (　) The Labor Standards Law sets working hours per week and companies cannot put a limit on overtime as they would like to.
4. (　) Some foreign workers in vocational training programs in Japan have ended up being karoshi victims.

B 音声を聴いて，次の英文の（　）内に適語を記入しなさい。　track 26

1. This area is (　) (　) crime.
2. Their wrongdoing will soon (　) (　).
3. Only children under 6 are (　) (　) the special service.
4. No workers were (　) (　) yesterday because the factory was closed.

C 和文に合うように，（　）内の語句を並べかえて英文をつくりなさい。

1. ボブは妻が自分の話を聞きながら疑わしげな目つきで自分を見ていることに気づいた。
   (him, his wife, doubtfully, while, Bob, at, caught, listening to, looking, him).

2. 公平さと信頼を維持するために，税法の抜け穴をふさぐことが急務である。
   (the tax law, to, fairness and reliability, urgent, it, in, is, loopholes, to, order, maintain, close, in).

3. 待機児童を減らすための政府の努力はほとんど成果を上げていない。
   (the waiting list, to, made, shorten, nurseries, have, headway, for, little, the government efforts).

4. 彼はほとんどなんでも一人でしょい込みがちである。
   (by, tends, almost anything, take, he, on, himself, to).

D 次の英語に相当する日本語を下から選び，記号で答えなさい。
1. part-timer （ ） 2. contractor （ ）
3. permanent position （ ） 4. managerial position （ ）
5. male-dominated （ ） 6. benefit （ ）
7. paid vacation （ ） 8. compensation （ ）
9. commit suicide （ ） 10. attempted suicide （ ）

a. 賠償金   b. 契約社員   c. 男性優位の
d. 非常勤で働く人 e. 自殺する   f. 管理職
g. 手当   h. 自殺未遂   i. 常勤職
j. 有給休暇

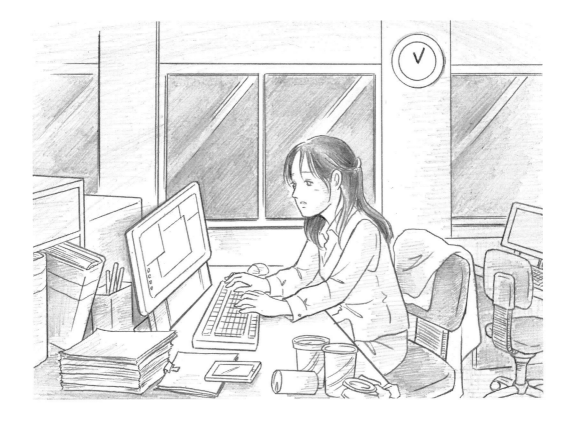

Unit 13 インドの肥満対策 ファーストフードに "肥満税"

India's Southern Kerala State Imposes "Fat Tax" on Fast Food

Voice of America, July 15, 2016

track 27

NEW DELHI — Customers in India's southern state of Kerala will have to dig deeper into their pockets each time they want to order a juicy burger, a cheese-laced pizza or other fast food such as doughnuts and tacos.

Vowing to combat rising levels of obesity—Kerala has the second highest levels of obesity in the country—the state government is imposing a 14.5 percent "fat tax" on fast foods sold by branded restaurants such as McDonald's and Pizza Hut.

India's first "fat tax"

Thomas Isaac, Kerala's finance minister, says he took the cue from a handful of countries that have experimented with similar taxes.

India's first such tax in the scenic, coastal state will only affect a small section of the country's increasingly affluent middle class, whose appetite for Western-style fast food has grown over the last decade-and-a-half. The measure has attracted national attention as India confronts growing levels of obesity.

Notes:

Kerala State／ケララ州（インド南西部の州） impose／課する New Delhi／ニューデリー（インドの首都） customer／客 dig deep into one's pocket／金を思い切って使う each time ～／～するたびに juicy／水分の多い, 汁の多い cheese-laced／チーズを織り込んだ A such as B／BのようなA vow to ～／～すると誓う combat／闘う obesity／（病的な）肥満 branded／商標のついた finance minister／財務大臣 take the cue from ～／～からヒントを得る a handful of ～／ひとつかみの～, 少量の～ experiment with ～／～の実験をする scenic／風光明媚な coastal／海岸沿いの affect／影響する increasingly／ますます affluent／裕福な appetite／食欲 last／すぐ前の decade-and-a-half／15年 measure／施策, 措置（通例は複数形） attract／引く attention／関心 confront／直面する

Critics question if it will actually deter people from getting their fix of junk food, and skeptics suspect it is probably meant to garner more revenue. Doctors and nutritionists, however, say it is a long overdue first step in that the country urgently needs to address its expanding waistlines.

Addressing obesity

With half of Indians under 25, worries center on young people in particular.

Anoop Misra, who heads the Center for Diabetes, Obesity and Cholesterol at Fortis Hospital in New Delhi, has watched with rising alarm as more and more people in their 20s and 30s walk into his clinic.

Strongly supporting the Kerala initiative, the doctor says, "We used to see diabetes 20 years back, diabetes in 50 or 40 years of age. Now we are seeing diabetes at 15 years of age, 18 years of age." Misra says he hopes the rest of the country will take the cue from the state's fat tax.

Global brands such as Pizza Hut, KFC and McDonald's have been ramping up their presence as the Indian fast food market grows exponentially while others such as Johnny Rockets, Burger King, Wendy's and Barcelos have begun making forays. Fast food chains have not commented on the tax so far.

Notes:
critic／批判する人　actually／実際　deter A from／～ing／Aに～することをやめさせる　fix／（習慣になって）やめられないもの　skeptic／疑い深い人　suspect (that) ～／～ではないかと思う　probably／おそらく　be meant to ～／～することになっている　garner／集める　revenue／租税収入　nutritionist／栄養学者　overdue／待望されている　in that ～／～という点において，～なので　urgently／緊急に　address／取り組む　expanding／広がりつつある　center on ～／～に集中する　in particular／特に　head／率いる　the Center for Diabetes, Obesity and Cholesterol at Fortis Hospital／フォルティス病院糖尿病・肥満・コレステロールセンター　with rising alarm／高まりつつある警鐘とともに　initiative／計画，新しい試み　used to ～／以前は～したものだ　the rest of ～／～の残り（の部分）　global brand／世界的ブランド　ramp up ～／～を増やす，強める　presence／存在（感）　exponentially／急激に　Johnny Rockets／ジョニー・ロケッツ（米国を本拠地とするハンバーガーチェーン店）　Barcelos／バルセロス（南アフリカ共和国を本拠地とするファーストフードチェーン店）　make a foray／進出する　so far／今までのところ

Money making initiative

The Kerala government has rejected suggestions that the tax aims to shore up its revenue, saying collections from such a tax will be small. Fast food outlets have a relatively small presence in the southern state compared to the north and the west.

Minister Isaac, who proposed the tax, says he simply sees it as a signal to move back to traditional healthy eating, a practice he says is "going out of fashion."

While acknowledging the need to target unhealthy food, many in Kerala point to local, deep-fried, highly popular local snacks and foods that are often sold at wayside stalls and restaurants. The owner of a café in Kerala's Kochi city, Isaac Alexander, says the format does not seem fair as it excludes such food.

One food that is eaten widely in Kerala is the "paratha." It is high in fat, high in refined flour; it is cheap. It can't be taxed because it is highly unorganized," he said.

Raising awareness, not taxing

Doctors and nutritionists agree that the tax needs to target a range of Indian snacks rich in trans fats that are sold throughout the country often on wayside stalls, as well as sugary drinks.

Notes:
make initiative／主導権をとる　reject／拒否する　suggestion／提案, 意見　aim to ～／～することを意図する　shore up ～／～を支える, ～を強化する　collection／徴収　a fast food outlet／ファーストフード店　relatively／比較的　compared to ～／～に比べて　propose／提案する　simply／単に　see A as B／AをBとみなす　a signal to ～／～するきっかけ　move back to ～／～に戻る　traditional／伝統的な　practice／習慣　out of fashion／すたれて　acknowledge／認識する　point to ～／～を指摘する　deep-fried／油をたっぷり使って揚げた　wayside／道端の　stall／屋台, 露店　Kochi city／コーチ市（ケララ州の都市）　format／構成, 様式　fair／公平な　exclude／除外する　"paratha"／「パラタ」（インド料理で, ロティの両面にギーを塗ってあぶったもの）　refined flour／精粉　unorganized／組織化されていない　raise awareness／意識を高める　agree／同意する　a range of ～／一連の～　rich in ～／～が豊富な　trans fat／トランス脂肪酸　throughout the country／国中　A as well as B／BだけでなくAも　sugary／砂糖のたくさん入った

"Is it enough? I don't think so. We need to go much beyond the burgers and the doughnuts and the French fries," says Sheela Krishnaswamy, a nutritionist who heads the Indian Dietetic Association in Bangalore. "It needs to be done more scientifically. At what percentage of fat in a food can the fat tax begin?"

A customer in New Delhi who is enjoying burgers with his family does not agree. Vijay Deoli says governments should focus on more urgent priorities like pollution.

"First you have to clear up the air, the water; many things are there," he said. "This is a small thing."

Others say the government should focus more on raising awareness about fast food instead of using taxes to influence people's choices.

"If you go by even developed countries, nowadays teachers or classrooms — they are training people, what should be eaten, and what should not be eaten," says IT engineer Gaurav Singh.

Denmark, for example, scrapped a fat tax when it found that customers were picking up their quota of high fat goods from other countries.

Health experts agree that raising awareness is critical; but, Dr. Misra feels that education alone is not doing the trick.

"As I see every day, people, they are well aware of what is good and what is bad, they will [still] most of the time veer towards bad eating," he said.

75　He compares the fat tax to a seatbelt law imposed some years back to force people to use seatbelts. "Everybody has a seatbelt. Previously nobody was wearing that. But now there is a fine. So a certain amount of regulation has to be brought in to change the habits of the people."

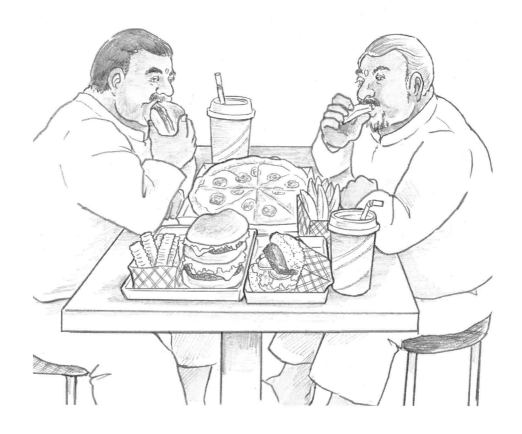

Notes:
compare A to B／AをBにたとえる　force A to ～／Aに無理やり～させる　previously／以前には　fine／罰金
a certain amount of ～／ある程度の～　regulation／規則　bring in ～／～を導入する　habit／習慣

練習問題

A 次の英文が本文の内容に一致する場合にはT，一致しない場合にはFを（　）内に記入しなさい。

1. (　) The state government imposes a "fat tax" on all goods sold by restaurants in Kerala.
2. (　) This fat tax will affect all people in Kerala.
3. (　) The head of the Center for Diabetes, Obesity and Cholesterol has watched many younger people in their 20's and 30's come to the hospital.
4. (　) Some people say that the aim of the fat tax is to collect more money.

B 音声を聴いて，次の英文の（　）内に適語を記入しなさい。　　track 28

1. Mary wanted to be a good cook and (　　) (　　) (　　) (　　) her grandmother.
2. The government will (　　) (　　) legislation to restrict the sale of guns.
3. Tom said that my idea was (　　) (　　) (　　).
4. Students should learn by themselves (　　) (　　) being taught everything.

C 和文に合うように，（　）内の語句を並べかえて英文をつくりなさい。

1. すべてのチームが世界一になることをめざしている。
   (in, all, the world, aim, become, to, the best, teams).

2. ジョンと同様に君も勤勉だね。
   (diligent, as, as, John, are, you, well).

3. 君はやってはならないことを知っておくべきだ。
   (aware, you, should, you, be, not, of, what, do, must).

4. 両親は彼に勉強することを強制した。
　　(forced, his, to, parents, him, study).

D 次の英語に相当する日本語を下から選び，記号で答えなさい。
1. appetite　　　　（　）　2. obesity　　　　　（　）
3. reject　　　　　（　）　4. nutritionist　　　（　）
5. diabetes　　　　（　）　6. pollution　　　　 （　）
7. exclude　　　　 （　）　8. accept　　　　　 （　）
9. include　　　　 （　）　10. regulation　　　 （　）

a. 汚染　　　　　b. 栄養学者　　　　c. 受け入れる
d. 糖尿病　　　　e. 食欲　　　　　　f. 除外する
g. 肥満　　　　　h. 規則　　　　　　i. 拒否する
j. 含む

Unit 14 高騰するアジアの医療費　その原因は？

WHO, Medical Experts, Warn of Rising Health Costs in Asia

Voice of America, February 06, 2017

track 29

BANGKOK — Asia faces a growing burden in treatment costs due to rising numbers of patients diagnosed with cancer, as well as those suffering from stroke and dementia over the next decade.

While Asia's economic progress has led to sharply lower levels of poverty, it has resulted in social and lifestyle changes ranging from diets to increasing urban pollution, that extract an increasing toll on communities.

The World Health Organization (WHO) says in Southeast Asia, late treatment of cancer results in 1.3 million deaths a year. The WHO says of the 8.8 million deaths from cancer annually, two thirds are in Africa and Asia.

Cancers, along with diabetes, cardiovascular and chronic lung diseases, were responsible for 40 million – or 70 percent of the world's 56 million deaths in 2015, the WHO said.

But globally treatment costs are rising. In 2015, the spending on cancer drugs rose by 11.5 percent to $107 billion, and is forecast to rise to $150 billion by 2020 – due largely to the expense of newer and more specialized

Notes:

WHO／世界保健機関 (the World Health Organization)　warn of ～／～を警告する　Bangkok／バンコク (タイ王国の首都)　face／直面する　burden／負担　treatment／治療　due to ～／～が原因で　rising numbers of ～／ますます多くの～　diagnose A with B／AをBと診断する　cancer／がん　A as well as B／BだけでなくAも　suffer from ～／～を患う　stroke／（脳）卒中　dementia／認知症　decade／10年間　economic／経済の　progress／発展, 成長　lead to ～／～につながる　poverty／貧困　result in ～／～の結果になる　diet／食事　urban／都市の　pollution／汚染　extract a toll on ～／～に被害をもたらす　annually／毎年, 1年間に　along with ～／～とともに　diabetes／糖尿病　cardiovascular／心（臓）血管の　chronic／慢性の　lung／肺　be responsible for ～／～の原因である　billion／10億　be forecast to ～／～すると予想される　expense／費用, 支出　specialized／専門的な, 特殊用途の

drugs.

The Boston Consulting Group said in a recent report the "cancer burden in developing countries is reaching pandemic proportions," seen as a leading cause of death in India with some 2.5 million patients. They forecast that India has "a chance of the disease rising five-fold by 2025."

China reported four million new cancer cases in 2016, with the national health bill set to soar "fourfold" to 12.7 trillion yuan ($1.84 trillion) by 2025, the consultants said.

Increased costs

Gregory Winter, a Cambridge University professor leading a research team in antibody engineering and modification technology for the treatment of degenerative diseases and several types of cancer, said while scientific progress has been made, treatment costs remain prohibitive for most populations.

"The challenges are much more in costs than in feasibility. I'm not saying everything is possible but I think in rolling treatments out to populations in general we will be struggling with cost problems. The cost of antibody treatment can be in the order of $15 to $75,000 per year and that's a lot for anybody," Winter said.

In China, reports say cancer patients and family care givers faced with the high cost of approved drugs lead to them seeking out generic drugs on the

Notes:
The Boston Consulting Group／ボストン・コンサルティング・グループ（米国に本社を置くコンサルティング会社）　developing country／発展途上国　pandemic／世界的に広がる　proportions／（複数形で）規模，程度　leading／第1位の，主要な　cause of death／死因　five-fold／5倍　national health bill／国民の医療費　set to ～／～しそうである　soar／急騰する　"fourfold"／「4倍」　trillion／兆　yuan／元（中国の通貨単位）　consultant／コンサルタント　Cambridge University／ケンブリッジ大学（英国の名門大学）　lead／率いる　antibody engineering and modification technology／抗体工学と修正技術　degenerative disease／変性疾患　prohibitive／手が出ないほど高い，法外な　feasibility／実行可能性　rolling treatments out to ～／～に治療を広める　in general／一般の　struggle with ～／～と戦う，～に取り組む　antibody treatment／抗体治療　in the order of ～／約～，およそ～　family care giver／家族介護者　approved drug／承認薬，認可薬　lead to A ～ing／Aを～する気にさせる（＝lead A to ～）　seek out ～／～を求める　generic drug／ジェネリック医薬品，後発医薬品

grey market to save costs. But the drugs may also be ineffective or fake.

Delays in China's drug approval process have sometimes led to drugs coming onto the Chinese market up to 10 years after they appeared in the U.S. market. Winter says a similar story of delay is also found in India, and says a solution may require some countries in Asia to "take more risks during the drug approval process."

"My own view is they should consider having a different drug approval process that is not so onerous and in return this should enable costs to be brought down for launching drugs in these markets," Winter said.

Stroke and dementia

Asia is also facing rising health costs in the treatment of growing numbers of patients in Asia affected by strokes and dementia.

The WHO, in a 2012 report, estimated globally 35.6 million people worldwide living with dementia – with the numbers forecast to reach 65.7 million in 2030 and 115.4 million by 2050.

The report said nearly 60 percent of the burden of dementia is concentrated in low and middle income countries, and is expected to increase in the years ahead.

"The catastrophic cost of care drives millions of households below the poverty line," with numbers and economic burden making it a "public health priority," the WHO said.

Notes:
grey market／非公式市場, 闇市場　ineffective／効き目がない　fake／偽の　delay／遅れ　drug approval process／薬品認可プロセス　up to ～／～まで　require A to ～／Aに～するように要求する　take risk／危険を冒す　onerous／やっかいな, わずらわしい　in return／代わりに　enable A to ～／Aが～できるようにする　bring down ～／～を下げる　launch／市場に出す, 発売する　growing numbers of ～／ますます多くの～　estimate／見積もる　live with ～／～を受け入れる, ～を我慢する　concentrate／集中する　in the years ahead／ここ何年かのうちに　catastrophic／破滅的な　drive／押しやる　millions of ～／何百万もの～　household／世帯　below the poverty line／貧困線以下の　"public health priority"／「公衆衛生対策上の優先課題」

Canadian, Vladimir Hachinski, a leading global specialist in stroke and vascular dementia, at the University of Western Ontario, said a growing bank of evidence links high rates of pollution, evident across Asia, with strokes and dementia.

In 2016, research by Valery Feigin, a director of the National Institute for Stroke and Applied Neurosciences at Auckland University of Technology, set a clear link between air pollution and strokes.

Air pollution

The research found air pollution in the form of fine particulate matter ranked seventh in terms of impact on healthy lives.

The findings found the impact of air pollution in causing harm to the lungs, heart and brain had previously been underestimated.

"This is a global problem because there are currents between the continents. There are currents in the atmosphere that carry air from one continent to another and also within the continents. So what happens in Beijing matters in Bangkok because the whole atmosphere is one in the biosphere," Hachinski said.

A recent report by the environmental group Greenpeace said as many as 1.2 million deaths occurred each year in India due to air pollution, just a fraction less than deaths from tobacco use.

Notes:
vascular dementia／血管性認知症　the University of Western Ontario／ウェスタンオンタリオ大学（カナダのオンタリオ州ロンドン市にある州立大学）　a growing bank of ～／ますます多くの～　link A with B／AとBを結びつける　evident／明白な　the National Institute for Stroke and Applied Neurosciences／（ニュージーランド）国立卒中および応用神経科学研究所　Auckland University of Technology／オークランド工科大学（ニュージーランドのオークランドにある国立大学）　between A and B／AとBの間　fine particulate matter／微粒子状物質　in terms of ～／～の点において　underestimate／過小評価する, 軽く見る　current／気流　continent／大陸　atmosphere／大気　from one continent to another／ひとつの大陸から別の大陸へ　Beijing／北京（中華人民共和国の首都）　matter／重要である, 問題となる　biosphere／生物圏　the environmental group Greenpeace／環境保護団体グリーンピース　as many as ～／～ほど多くの　fraction／少し　less than ～／～より少ない

In China, cities such as Beijing continued to face regular bouts of choking smog during the current winter season amid high reported levels of harmful particle matter.

Studies indicate that smog leads to more than a million premature deaths in China each year, cutting life expectancy by two to five years.

Hachinski said Asia has to confront the issues of pollution as it faces a significant rise in pollution-induced strokes, as well as dementia in increasingly aging populations.

"At the rate we are going, we cannot afford more patients having strokes, more patients having dementia – particularly Asia – 61 percent of the world's population is in Asia."

"In some countries like China, stroke is the leading cause of death and in Japan, of course, you have an aging population, you have high rates of stroke and dementia," he said.

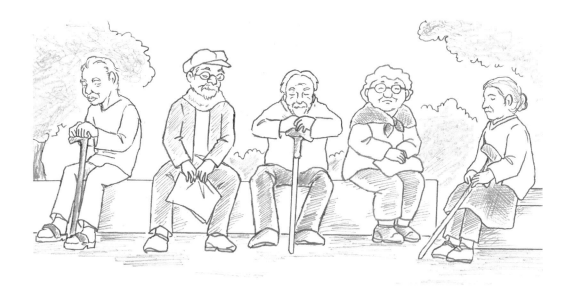

Notes:

A such as B／BのようなA　bout／ひとしきり，短い期間　choking smog／窒息させるようなスモッグ　amid ～／～に囲まれて　particle matter／粒子状物質　more than ～／～より多い　premature death／早死に　life expectancy／余命　confront／直面する，立ち向かう　issue／問題(点)　significant／重要な　pollution-induced／汚染によって引き起こされた　aging／高齢の　afford／（金・時間などに）余裕がある

練習問題

A 本文の内容に合うように，各英文の（ ）に入るもっとも適当な語句をそれぞれ1つずつ選びなさい。

1. Asia faces a growing burden in treatment costs due to (rising, equal, decreasing) numbers of patients diagnosed with cancer.

2. Cancer patients and family care givers faced with the high cost of approved drugs lead to them seeking out (over-the-counter, generic, wonder) drugs on the grey market to save costs.

3. (Denials, Acceptance, Delays) in China's drug approval process have sometimes led to drugs coming onto the Chinese market up to 10 years after they appeared in the U.S. market.

4. The catastrophic cost of care drives millions of households below the (sea level, poverty line, freezing point).

B 音声を聴いて，次の英文の（ ）内に適語を記入しなさい。　track 30
1. The young lady was (　　　)(　　　) AIDS.
2. My father is (　　　)(　　　) diabetes.
3. Smoking (　　　)(　　　)(　　　) her lung cancer.
4. Many people worldwide are (　　　)(　　　) dementia.

C 和文に合うように，（ ）内の語句を並べかえて英文をつくりなさい。
1. バランスの取れていない食事は，しばしば生活習慣病を引き起こす。
   (diets, diseases, result, unbalanced, often, in, lifestyle-related).

2. 彼は10年間にわたっていくつかの病気と闘ってきている。
   (has, struggling, he, a, been, with, decade, several, over, diseases).

3. ますます多くの生徒たちが東京の大学に入学したがっている。
   (of, like, growing, would, universities in Tokyo, enter, numbers, to, students).

4. 脳卒中が中国では死因の第1位である。
   (is, of, China, cause, the, stroke, leading, in, death).

D 次の英語に相当する日本語を下から選び，記号で答えなさい。

1. chronic disease （　） 2. degenerative disease （　）
3. incurable disease （　） 4. respiratory disease （　）
5. preventable disease （　） 6. acute disease （　）
7. infectious disease （　） 8. sexually transmitted disease （　）
9. inherited disease （　） 10. congenital disease （　）

> a. 予防できる病気　　　b. 性感染症　　　c. 先天性疾患
> d. 慢性疾患　　　　　　e. 感染症　　　　f. 遺伝性疾患
> g. 急性疾患　　　　　　h. 変性疾患　　　i. 呼吸器疾患
> j. 不治の病

Unit 15 麻薬使用に対する世界各国の取り組み

> ## UN Hears Major Differences on Global Approach to Drug Use
>
> Voice of America, April 21, 2016
> Associated Press

🔊 track 31

UNITED NATIONS — Jamaica defended its decriminalization of possession of small amounts of marijuana. Iran said it seized 620 tons of different types of drugs last year and is helping protect the world from "the evils of addiction." Cuba opposed the legalization of drugs or declaring them
5 harmless.

The first U.N. General Assembly special session to address global drug policy in nearly 20 years heard major differences on the approach to drug use on its second day on Wednesday.

On the liberalization side, Canada's Health Minister Jane Philpott
10 announced that the government will introduce legislation to legalize marijuana next spring. She said (1)Canada will ensure that marijuana is kept out children's hands, and will address the devastating consequences of drugs and drug-related crimes.

Jamaica's Foreign Minister Kamina Johnson Smith told delegates that the
15 government amended the Dangerous Drugs Act last year to give tickets for possession of less than two ounces of cannabis instead (2   ) making it a felony offense, and to legalize the sacramental use of marijuana by Rastafarians. It also established provisions for the medical, scientific and therapeutic uses of the plant, she said.

20 Smith said (3)Jamaica is finalizing a five-year national drug plan including programs to reduce demand for drugs, provide for early intervention and treatment of drug users, and promote rehabilitation and social reintegration.

98

Michael Botticelli, director of the White House Office of National Drug Control Policy, stressed that (4)"law enforcement efforts should focus on criminal organizations—not on people with substance use disorders who need treatment and recovery support services."

He called for drug policies in every country to address the needs of underserved groups including women and children, indigenous people, prisoners, and lesbians, gays, bisexual and transgender people.

On the tough enforcement side, Indonesia's Ambassador Rachmat Budiman said "a zero-tolerance approach" is needed to suppress and eliminate the scourge of drugs.

He said drug trafficking rings are using new "psychoactive substances" and the Internet to penetrate all levels of society, including the young generation, and pose "a serious threat which requires extraordinary efforts."

Like Indonesia, Iran imposes the death penalty on drug traffickers.

Iran's Justice Minister Abdulreza Rahmani Fazli told the high-level meeting that the Islamic Republic (5)[drug traffickers, in, of, armed, spent, against, dollars, billions, has, its campaign].

He said Iran is ready to host an international conference on countering drugs and drug-related crimes along the Balkan route, one of the two main heroin trafficking corridors linking opium-producing Afghanistan to the huge markets of Russia and Western Europe. It usually goes through Pakistan to Iran, Turkey, Greece and Bulgaria across southeastern Europe to the Western European market, and has an annual market value of some $28 billion, according to the U.N. Office of Drugs and Crime known (6) UNODC.

Fazli said the conference, in collaboration (7) the UNODC and countries on the route, would tackle ways to combat drug-related money laundering and detect drug trafficking ringleaders.

Cuba's Justice Minister Maria Esther Reus Gonzalez asked how the world couldn't be worried when the world drug problem has become "deeper and more intensified" with 246 million people using illicit drugs, according (8) UNODC.

"(9)It will be really difficult to solve the problems of mass production of and trafficking in drugs from the South, if the majority demand from the North is not eliminated," she warned.

Reus Gonzalez also warned that legalizing drugs won't solve the problem either and will only open "more dangerous gaps for the stability of our nations." (10)She reiterated "Cuba's absolutely commitment to achieving societies free of illicit drugs."

Notes:

UN／国際連合（the United Nations） Associated Press／AP通信社（米国の大手通信社） defend／擁護する decriminalization／非犯罪化, 刑罰の軽減化 possession／所持 marijuana／マリファナ, 大麻 seize／押収する "the evils of addiction"／「中毒の弊害」 oppose／反対する legalization／合法化 declare／断言する General Assembly special session／（国際連合の）特別総会 address／取り組む liberalization／自由化 Health Minister／保健大臣, 厚生相 introduce legislation／法案を提出する legalize／合法化する ensure／確実に～になるようにする devastating／壊滅的な consequence／結果 crime／犯罪 Foreign Minister／外務大臣, 外相 delegate／代表 amend／（法律などを）修正する the Dangerous Drug Act／危険薬物法 give tickets for ～／～に対する違反切符を切る less than ～／～より少ない ounce／オンス（約28.35グラム） cannabis／カンナビス, インド大麻 felony／重罪 offense／犯罪 sacramental／聖餐用の Rastafarian／ラスタファリアン（ラスタファリ運動の実践者） establish／定める, 規定する provision／条項 therapeutic／治療上の finalize／完成させる reduce／減少させる intervention／介入 treatment／治療 social reintegration／社会復帰 director of the White House Office of National Drug Control Policy／ホワイトハウス国家薬物取締政策局長官 law enforcement／法の執行 criminal organization／犯罪組織 substance use disorder／物質使用障害 call for A to ～／Aが～することを求める underserved／サービスが行き届いていない indigenous people／先住民 prisoner／囚人 lesbian／レズビアン gay／ゲイ bisexual／バイセクシュアルの transgender／トランスジェンダーの tough／強硬な, 断固たる ambassador／大使 "a zero-tolerance approach"／「容認ゼロアプローチ」 suppress／抑圧する eliminate／排除する scourge／災難, 苦難 trafficking ring／密売組織 "psychoactive substance"／「精神作用物質」 penetrate／浸透する, 入り込む pose／引き起こす, もたらす a serious threat／深刻な脅威 extraordinary／並はずれた, 驚くほどの impose／科する death penalty／死刑 drug trafficker／麻薬密売人 Justice Minister／司法大臣, 法相 high-level meeting／高官レベルの会議 Islamic Republic／イスラム共和国 armed／武装した billion／十億 campaign／軍事行動 be ready to ～／進んで～する host／主催する conference／会議 counter／対抗する, 阻止する the Balkan route／バルカン諸国ルート heroin／ヘロイン trafficking corridor／密売回廊地帯 opium-producing／アヘンを生産する the U. N. Office of Drugs and Crime／国連薬物・犯罪事務所（略語はUNODC） tackle／取り組む money laundering／マネーローンダリング, 資金洗浄 detect／みつけ出す drug trafficking ringleader／麻薬密売の首謀者 deep／深刻な, 複雑な intensified／激化した illicit drug／不法麻薬, 違法薬物 the South／（アジア・アフリカ・中南米などの）発展途上国 majority demand／大部分の需要

the North／先進国 stability／安定 reiterate／繰り返す absolutely／絶対的に，断固として commitment／積極的関与，献身 achieve／達成する free of ～／～のない，～のおそれがない

練習問題

A 本文中の (2) (6) (7) (8) に適語を入れなさい（音声を参考にしてもよい）。
(2) (　　　　) (6) (　　　　　) (7) (　　　　　　) (8) (　　　　　　　)

B (5) が「武装した麻薬密売人に対する運動に何十億ドルも費やしてきた」という意味になるように [　　　] 内の語句を並べかえなさい（音声を参考にしてもよい）。

C 下線部 (1) (3) (4) (9) (10) を日本語に直しなさい。
(1)

(3)

(4)

(9)

(10)

D 次の説明に合う語を英文中から選びなさい。

(11) the condition of being unable to stop taking or doing something harmful
(   )

(12) something that someone does that is against the law (   )

(13) medical care for an illness or injury (   )

(14) an official who represents their own country in a foreign country
(   )

(15) a meeting for discussion or exchange of opinions (   )

Review (Unit 11〜Unit 14)

A 英文の（　）内に入る語を下から選んで記入し，英文を日本語に直しなさい。

1. What prompted you (   ) give up your job? (Unit 11)

2. He was forced to flee the country, leaving (   ) his wife and daughters. (Unit 12)

3. I went (   ) the store on my way home and got some food. (Unit 13)

4. The farmer offered us food (   ) return for our work. (Unit 14)

> by,　behind,　in,　to

B 和文に合うように，（　）内の語句を並べかえて英文をつくりなさい。

1. 今週末にしたいことが特に何かありますか？ (Unit 11)
   (do, there, you'd like to, particular, this weekend, in, anything, is) ?

2. いま十分にお金を貯めておけば快適に退職できるだろう。(Unit 12)
   (to, now, you, retire comfortably, saving, enable, enough money, will).

3. 高額なので若い夫婦たちは家を買うことを思いとどまっている。(Unit 13)
   (young couples, high prices, buying, are, from, houses, deterring).

4. 乗客はシートベルト着用を求められている。(Unit 14)
   (belts, required, seat, are, to, passengers, wear).

C 次の英語に相当する日本語を下から選び，記号で答えなさい。

1. awareness   (   )   2. institution   (   )
3. representative (   )   4. solution   (   )
5. right   (   )   6. stroke   (   )
7. revenue   (   )   8. poverty   (   )
9. atmosphere   (   )   10. biosphere   (   )

> a. 脳卒中   b. 生物圏   c. 解決
> d. 大気   e. 租税収入 f. 意識
> g. 貧困   h. 代表者   i. 施設
> j. 権利

編著者紹介

田中　芳文（たなか　よしふみ）
1985年　岡山大学大学院教育学研究科（英語教育専攻）修了
島根県立大学大学院看護学研究科・看護学部教授　などを経て，
2018年4月より　島根県立大学人間文化学部教授

NDC 490　　109p　　26cm

やさしい英語ニュースで学ぶ　現代社会と健康

2018年2月23日　第1刷発行
2023年2月15日　第3刷発行

編著者	田中芳文（たなかよしふみ）
発行者	髙橋明男
発行所	株式会社　講談社 〒112-8001　東京都文京区音羽2-12-21 　　販　売　（03）5395-4415 　　業　務　（03）5395-3615
編　集	株式会社　講談社サイエンティフィク 　代表　堀越俊一 〒162-0825　東京都新宿区神楽坂2-14　ノービィビル 　　編　集　（03）3235-3701
印刷所	株式会社ＫＰＳプロダクツ
製本所	株式会社国宝社

落丁本・乱丁本は，購入書店名を明記のうえ，講談社業務宛にお送りください．送料小社負担にてお取替えいたします．なお，この本の内容についてのお問い合わせは，講談社サイエンティフィク宛にお願いいたします．定価はカバーに表示してあります．

© Yoshifumi Tanaka, 2018

本書のコピー，スキャン，デジタル化等の無断複製は著作権法上での例外を除き禁じられています．本書を代行業者等の第三者に依頼してスキャンやデジタル化することはたとえ個人や家庭内の利用でも著作権法違反です．

JCOPY 〈(社)出版者著作権管理機構委託出版物〉
複写される場合は，その都度事前に(社)出版者著作権管理機構（電話 03-5244-5088, FAX 03-5244-5089, e-mail: info@jcopy.or.jp）の許諾を得てください．

Printed in Japan
ISBN978-4-06-155633-1